FIT

TO BE

Bride

FIT
TO BE
Bride

THE COMPLETE
WEDDING WORKOUT

BONNE MARCUS

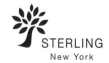

STERLING
New York

Dedicated to my husband Lawrence,
the love of my life.

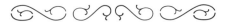

STERLING
New York

An Imprint of Sterling Publishing
1166 Avenue of the Americas
New York, NY 10036

Text © 2015 by Bonne Marcus
Illustrations © 2015 by Sterling Publishing Co., Inc.
Illustrations by Nina Matsumoto

ISBN 978-1-4549-1519-5

Distributed in Canada by Sterling Publishing
c/o Canadian Manda Group, 664 Annette Street
Toronto, Ontario, Canada M6S 2C8
Distributed in the United Kingdom by GMC Distribution Services
Castle Place, 166 High Street, Lewes, East Sussex, England BN7 1XU
Distributed in Australia by Capricorn Link (Australia) Pty. Ltd.
P.O. Box 704, Windsor, NSW 2756, Australia

For information about custom editions, special sales, and premium
and corporate purchases, please contact Sterling Special Sales at
800-805-5489 or specialsales@sterlingpublishing.com.

Manufactured in Canada

2 4 6 8 10 9 7 5 3 1

www.sterlingpublishing.com

CONTENTS

A Fitness Fairy Tale

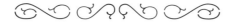

Once upon a time, there was a beautiful princess who snagged a handsome Prince Charming. They got engaged and set a date. When the time came for her to pick her wedding gown, the one she chose fit her to perfection. She had a "princess" figure, so endless fittings were not needed. The princess floated to her big day on a cushion of air. Now you, too, have found your soul mate, and will be looking for the perfect dress.

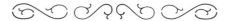

Unlike the beautiful princess (who, by the way, lived in a fairy tale, where scales don't exist), you may be feeling the need to get in shape. To look like the princess on your wedding day, put down the storybooks and jump on the treadmill. If you'd like to tone up certain body parts, like your arms and your back, you must pick up the weights yourself.

The princess had servants—everything from cook to royal dresser. Half the allure of the whole princess thing is the perks and support, right? Would she have looked so good having done her own hair? I don't think so. But even Cinderella needed a fairy godmother to get it together, and that whole look didn't even last a night.

So, what can *you* do? This is where I come in. Looking perfect is not a job for one person, so consider me your fairy godtrainer. I will help you become a princess bride, and there doesn't have to be a midnight transformation back to the old you. *What?* Don't all personal trainers have a magic wand?

By the way, there is a moral to this fable. While your big day may give you reason to get in shape, the fact that your overall quality of life will improve is the real benefit. Living a longer, healthier, and happier life with the person you most cherish is reason enough to organize your time so that your body feels as complete as your heart.

HOW TO USE THIS BOOK

Consider this book your portable personal trainer. It is designed to coach you through getting in shape for your wedding and beyond. Chapter 1 covers the bridal body basics: cardio, strength, and flexibility training guidelines to give you a healthy foundation for achieving your fitness goals.

Since we know it's all about the dress, your workout should be structured around what you're wearing. In Chapter 3, my wedding dress workouts will help you improve the assets that your particular dress will show off.

The Down-the-Aisle workout in Chapter 4 is designed to get you the body you desire in 12 weeks. It combines quick agility-based cardio bursts with innovative and effective strength-training exercises that work together to boost metabolism, burn calories, and reshape your body.

Chapter 5 is all about your honeymoon. The cardio comparison in this chapter will help you decide which cardio is best for improving your endurance, and I've included a high-intensity interval cardio workout to build stamina.

No woman can stay fit by sweat alone, and the bride's healthy-eating guide in Chapter 6 covers everything you need to know about nutrition.

Finally, get tips on how to maintain your wedding-trained physique well after the nuptials in Chapter 7. Let's get started today—and before you know it, you'll be "fit to be bride"!

CHAPTER 1

A Marriage
of the Mind
and Body

ow many times have I heard someone say, "If I just started running, I would look great," or "I don't need to lift weights; I'm a girl," or "I don't have time to stretch"? A balanced and effective fitness program has to cover all the essentials of exercise and good health. Just like you wouldn't buy a dress on a hunch, neither should you begin a fitness program without first understanding what fitness is and making assumptions about what you should and should not do. There is a trinity of fitness: cardiovascular fitness, muscle strength, and flexibility. All of these elements are essential to keep your body strong and in balance, and understanding the whys and hows of each part of the trinity will ensure success.

Here's the perfect example: You have just returned from your bridal shower. Your mother-in-law-to-be has given you a box with service for eight of your preferred formal china from Tiffany's. Nice gift! Can you lift it with ease and carry it up to your apartment on the fourteenth floor? Did I mention the elevator isn't working? Are you breathing easily as you reach the tenth floor, or is your breathing labored? Now you've made it to your apartment. Catch your breath. You want to proudly display the china. Can you reach the top shelf of your antique cabinet with ease? Are you getting the picture?

CARDIOVASCULAR ACTIVITY

Cardiovascular (aerobic) exercise is defined as any repetitive activity using the larger muscle groups in your body that elevates your heart rate over a sustained period. Running, bicycling, and stair climbing—and if you're real daring, kayaking—are a few examples! If the sight of your fiancé makes your heart rate rise and you become short of breath, bear in mind, this does not count. It's ironic that cardio exercise affects the body a lot like being in love. So why don't more people love to exercise?

The secret to a successful cardio workout is finding an activity you love. Sorry, sex doesn't count (although if it's done long enough, you can burn a few extra calories). You don't want to drag yourself to the gym and then be miserable over every step you take on the StairMaster, so don't do it. You are guaranteed to burn out, so be creative. If no one cardio workout

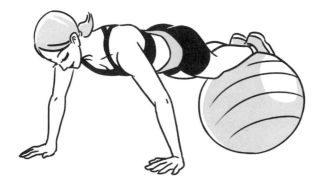

grabs you, then vary your routine. Zumba, jogging, Spinning, using the elliptical machine, rowing, African dance—whatever gets you moving, do it! (See Chapter 4 for more ideas.) You don't have to *love* an exercise, but you do have to like it enough to do it regularly.

No, we are not talking about *that*. What makes exercise effective is the *frequency, intensity, and duration* of your workout, also known as the FIT principle.

In terms of frequency, it's clear that if you exercise sporadically, you will see little to no results. Understanding how to measure intensity will help you determine the ideal duration. Pushing yourself too hard can lead to injury, inhibit progress, and increase the odds of giving up from burnout. On the other hand, if you do not push yourself hard enough, you will miss out on the benefits of cardiovascular exercise, such as losing weight, burning fat, and lowering blood pressure.

The simplest way to monitor how hard you are working is called the talk test. Can you carry on a conversation while you are exercising? If you are terribly short of breath and can't even say, "Stop this treadmill—I need to get off!" then it's time to lower the intensity and slow down. If, however, you can talk at length about your wedding plans or worse yet, text on your cell phone, you *need to put down the phone* and pick up the pace a little.

Using the Rate of Perceived Exertion (RPE) is another great way to gauge intensity. Use the following scale, based on the Borg Scale developed by Swedish physiologist Gunnar Borg.

RPE 1–2: Very easy, you can talk at length about your wedding

RPE 3: Easy, you can talk about the wedding with almost no effort

RPE 4: Moderately easy, you can talk about the wedding comfortably

RPE 5: Moderate, it requires some effort to talk about the wedding

RPE 6: Moderately hard, requires a bit more effort to talk about the wedding

RPE 7: Difficult, requires a lot more effort to talk about the wedding

RPE 8: Very Difficult, it requires a maximum effort to talk about the wedding

RPE 9–10: Maximum effort, you CAN'T talk about the wedding

Since you want results in 12 weeks, aim for 45 minutes of cardiovascular exercise a day, 4 to 5 times per week, at a moderate to difficult intensity (think 6 to 8 on a scale of 1 to 10). For the busy bride, aim for 30 minutes a day, 3 times a week, working at a higher intensity (think 8, maybe 9, on a scale of 1 to 10).

Beginners and super busy brides, don't be discouraged; it does not have to be all or nothing. Ten minutes 2 to 4 times a day will be a great way to get started or stay on track on really hectic days. In chapter 4, learn how to maximize your aerobic workouts with cross-training and high-intensity interval training. But remember, a bride's body does not get toned by cardio alone!

STRENGTH TRAINING

So many brides forget resistance training. Why strength train? While cardio exercise is a great way to shed excess body fat, it will not change your shape. If you are shaped like a large pear and you are only doing cardio, you become a smaller pear! To really fit into the wedding dress of your dreams, you must do some resistance training. This can be weight lifting, Pilates, some forms of yoga, and calisthenics.

In fact, regular weight training may burn more calories and fat than aerobic training. How? Strength training with weights increases your muscle mass (which does not mean you'll get bigger), and the more muscle you have, the higher your basal metabolic rate, or BMR, will be. This is a good thing. The BMR is the rate at which your body burns calories when you're at rest. The higher the BMR, the more calories you burn. So when you work out with weights, you're not just burning calories; you're turning your body into a more efficient calorie-burning machine, *and* you're changing the shape of your body!

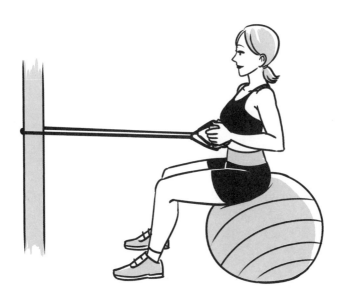

The intensity of your workout and your current fitness level will determine the amount of time needed for proper recovery. This point is particularly important for brides who exercise infrequently or haven't exercised in a while. For the Down-the-Aisle workout in Chapter 4, allow at least 48 hours between strength-training sessions and try to do it 2 to 3 times a week.

If you are short on time, look at the wedding dress workouts in Chapter 3 and do one a day. The dress you selected will be a combination of styles (for example: sweetheart neckline and form fitted). You may also split up the exercises by styles. If your dress plunges in front or back, do the chest and back workout on Mondays. Then do the halter top (upper back and shoulders) and strapless (arms and shoulders) gowns on Wednesdays and the sheath and form-fitted dress workout (booty, legs, and abs) on Fridays. You would rest on Tuesday, Thursday, and Saturday. If, however, you decide to work out on Tuesday, Thursday, and Saturday, make the rest days Wednesday, Friday, and Sunday or Monday. You may also decide to do 3 days in a row and take a day off in between. You can follow whatever schedule works best for you. Do not neglect any one body part just because it does not reflect your dress. Make sure to work each body part at least once a week.

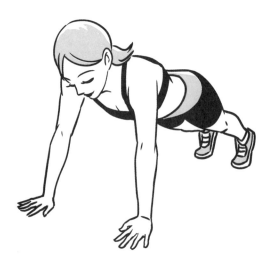

Learning the basics of strength training and proper form for performing exercises correctly will allow for a lifetime love affair with weight training.

You had to learn the names of your groom's family and friends to make a good impression, right? Well, improve your relationship with fitness (and get the best results from your workout) by learning the names of your major muscle groups. Understanding how each one operates and applying the following strength-training guidelines will ensure a safe and effective fitness plan. My mission is not only to make you fit for your wedding but to also give you a healthy foundation in exercise.

■ Warming Up

What exactly does warming up do for you? It helps limit muscle damage. Like starting up a car that has sat in a lot overnight, a warm-up increases the temperature in your cold muscles and in the tissue that connects muscle to bone. Warmer muscles and joints are more pliable and are less likely to tear. Always warm up your muscles and joints with 5 to 10 minutes of aerobic exercise.

■ Proper Form

Keeping your body beautifully poised and still through wedding picture after wedding picture ensures you will have a visual testament to match the memories. Fitness posture is just as important. Proper form is necessary to prevent injury and isolate the muscles the exercise is designed to work. Form always takes precedence over the amount of weight you lift: If you can't complete an entire set with perfect form, you're lifting too much and not getting the full benefit from your workout.

■ Don't Forget the Core

Do you want to be to be able stand for all your wedding pictures without suffering? The abdominal muscles, along with your hip, buttocks, and back muscles, are defined as your core. They are the initiators of movement, stabilizers of other muscles, and decelerators (they slow down movement).

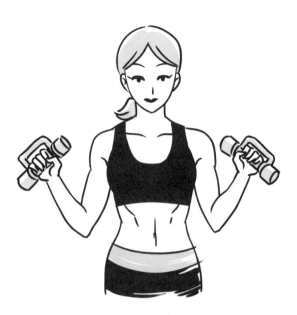

Developing your core muscles is vital to any long-term fitness program. And in fact, a strong core improves your quality of life in general and can support the strengthening of your entire body. Core-specific exercises encourage proper form, so save them for last. Core strength is needed in stabilizing your body during all activities and exercises.

■ *Rest*

As much as I love the adrenaline rush of exercise, to prevent overtraining and promote good health, one full day of rest every week is essential, and by rest, I mean total inertia. Don't think of a day off as a day wasted; it's necessary.

Rest is essential in an exercise program. No matter your skill level, each body has its limits. So you have to know the difference between "feeling the burn" and "burning out." Without adequate rest, strength gains diminish, motivation drops, and risk of injury or illness increases.

Always listen to your body. Cut back when it tells you to. Rest is something we all take for granted. With all you have on your list of to-dos for the wedding, it may become more difficult to fit in the wall-to-wall workouts and stay on track. That's okay, because sometimes the best thing you can do for your body is nothing at all.

No less important than strength training and cardiovascular exercise, flexibility is the most overlooked component of fitness. A regular stretching routine will help improve your posture and your overall ability to exercise.

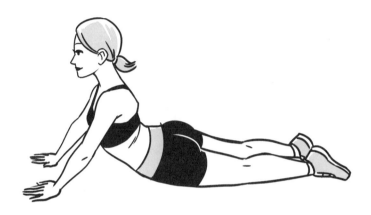

Notice your posture when you're working out and when you are at rest. If your neck and trapezius muscles (one of the major muscles of the back responsible for moving and stabilizing the shoulder blade as well extending the head at the neck) are tight (and whose wouldn't be with the stress of planning a wedding?), your head will angle forward. If your shoulders and chest are too tight, your shoulders will round inward. Imagine how that would look in your strapless gown. Not very flattering! Stretching will help avoid muscle imbalances, which can often lead to pulled muscles, injury, and even poor posture. As you stretch, your range of motion increases, allowing you to perform easy tasks, like bending down to pull up your dress to reveal your garter, or more challenging ones, like the limbo (wink, wink) on your honeymoon vacation in Hawaii. But beware of pitfalls by following these simple rules of stretching:

1. Never stretch a cold muscle. Always warm up before you stretch. Warming up, or encouraging blood flow through the tissue, loosens muscles and allows them to operate more efficiently and effectively.

2. Stretch at the end of every workout.

3. Stretch all of your muscles, not just the ones you've used in your workout.

4. Ease into a stretch. Start by spending 10 to 30 seconds in the *easy stretch*. Go to the point where you feel a mild tension, and relax as you hold the stretch. The tension will subside gradually. If it does not, back off until you are comfortable. As you become comfortable in the easy stretch, slowly move a fraction of an inch farther until you feel a mild tension, and hold that position for 10 to 30 seconds. Again, ease off slightly if you feel discomfort.

5. Never bounce. Ballistic stretching causes the muscles to contract and tighten. Ease into the stretch and hold it for the entire time.

6. Breathe consistently. As you stretch, your breathing should be slow, rhythmic, and controlled. Do not hold your breath while stretching. If a stretch position inhibits normal breathing, ease up.

WHERE DO I BEGIN?

Before we embark on this fitness journey together, check with your physician. It's always a good idea to consult a doctor before starting any new health regimen. Getting started is never easy. I remember a lot of false starts before I got it together fitness-wise. Plan your workout schedule like you plan your wedding: Give yourself as much time as possible to get ready for your wedding day. The biggest mistake I've seen brides make is waiting too long to start a fitness program.

Know what you want and have detailed goals in mind. Don't just proclaim your desire to lose weight. Make it specific. How much do you want to lose? What clothing size do you want to fit into? By what date? What waist size do you want? How many inches do you want to lose? I make sure that I write all my goals down in order to commit to them. Use a journal or a workout log, and record your goals and review them regularly. You will find a space to record your workouts and goals at the end of this book.

Keep in mind that these changes need to be realistic. If you are a size 16, it's unrealistic and self-defeating to tell yourself that you'll fit into a size 4 in 2 months. It's more probable that dropping one or two sizes is a realistic goal, with more sizes to lose as you keep on working on your goals.

Give yourself at least 3 to 6 months, and aim to lose one to two pounds per week.

WHAT YOU'LL NEED

You need only a few items that can be purchased at any sporting goods store or ordered online. For example, I like www.performbetter.com.

DUMBBELLS

Dumbbells are one of the most versatile exercise tools you can own. With one pair of dumbbells, you can do hundreds of exercises. Pick out three sets in weights that you consider light, medium, and heavy. As your strength grows, so will your dumbbell collection.

Portable, cheap, and convenient—a jump rope provides no excuses! It's a fantastic way to burn calories and lose weight. You can jump at your own level of intensity for any length of time almost anywhere.

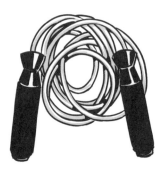

GLIDING DISC

This Frisbee-shaped disc will transform exercise movements into smooth, graceful lines of flowing motion. These are so much fun that they take the *work* out of workouts!

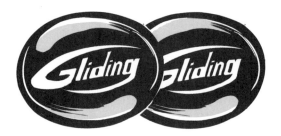

RESISTANCE BAND OR TUBING

This option is as multifunctional as dumbbells. Resistance bands are large rubber bands made in a variety of shapes and degrees of resistance. They are one of the most inexpensive types of equipment you'll ever buy. You may even consider packing one in your suitcase when you go on your honeymoon!

Created by personal trainer Marc Lebert, this has fast become a staple piece of equipment that I use with all my clients. It is simply a pair of hurdle-like bars that work the arms, chest, back, and core muscles like no other piece of equipment can, using your own body weight as resistance. You can order them at www.lebertfitness.com.

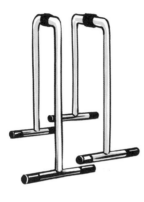

BODY BAR

Like resistance bands and dumbbells, the Body Bar is multifunctional and comes in a variety of sizes and weights.

STABILITY BALL

The stability ball is one of my favorite pieces of equipment. Exercises on the ball promote body awareness, improve balance and coordination, and reinforce proper spinal alignment. It's ideal for stretching, strengthening, and toning exercises, and when used with dumbbells, Kettlebells, or tubing, provides an added challenge to your exercise routine.

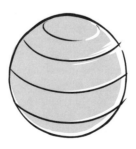

TIPS TO STAY MOTIVATED

BELIEVE IT CAN HAPPEN: Make certain you truly believe that you can achieve the goals you set for yourself. See yourself achieving those goals. You must believe you can do it . . . and are worth it. Visualize every change you want to make to your appearance, your eating habits, and your workouts. Look in the mirror and focus on the specific changes you want to make. Plan your workouts—run through a workout in your head on the way to the gym so the process is already ingrained in your psyche by the time you get there. Visualizing your plans makes it easier to follow through with them. Telling yourself you can do it gives you a positive attitude and goes a long way in helping you make plans a reality.

COMMIT TO THE PLAN, THEN GO FOR IT: Okay . . . you've got your workout plan with your specific goals, you've been visualizing your success, and you're telling yourself you can do it. Now what? *Follow through.* All the wishful thinking in the world is not going to make your goals happen. Here's where you must take action and "just do it." Realize that you don't have to *love* exercise for it to work—if you follow through with your well-devised plan, it *will* work.

FOCUS ON THE PROCESS: Rome wasn't built in a day. Concentrate on what you can do day by day and understand that it is all about the process rather than the destination. Long-term fitness goals are just that: long term. Programs that offer "quick results in just 2 weeks" usually sacrifice quality for empty promises to get your money. Understand that your goals will take committed, small steps over time. Remind yourself that your actions are cumulative; ask yourself, "Will what I am about to do help me achieve my goals?" Make positive, consistent choices.

ACCEPT SETBACKS, THEN REGROUP: One skipped workout, one not-so-good meal, or one too many office cookies is not going to destroy your fitness and health goals. Keep in mind that you'll slip up occasionally, but don't beat yourself up over it. Instead, focus on what happened: Did I skip exercise because I didn't plan my day appropriately? Could I have scaled back the workout instead of missing one entirely? Did my eating go down the drain on a particular day because I didn't pack my lunch like I had planned? Be realistic about your situation and then make changes accordingly.

MAKE IT A GROUP EFFORT: Boost your motivation to exercise by doing it with your bridesmaids.

RETAIL THERAPY: Nothing motivates me more than a new pair of sneakers and a new workout outfit!

EXERCISE FIRST THING IN THE MORNING: This has been a hugely successful tip for many of my clients: *Set the alarm clock 30 minutes early.* You will feel great knowing you have completed your workout. It will energize you for the rest of the day. You've done it and you won't have any reason to make excuses later. Sound undoable? Well, I ask you to try it for 21 days. (This is how many days it takes to create a habit.)

FINALLY, DON'T JUDGE YOURSELF: This process takes planning and work, but it's all worth it! Keep in mind the goal is more than just your measurements or size for the big day. While your wedding day may give you a reason to get in shape, living a longer, healthier, and happier life with the person you love is still the most important reason. Practice those vows . . . "For better, for worse, in weight gain and in thin times."

NOW IT'S TIME TO GET TO WORK!

CHAPTER 2

*Diary
of a
Fit Bride*

To help you focus, keep a workout diary. Include notes or reflections on how you feel after you've exercised. For example, say you ran 4 miles on the treadmill at 6.0 miles per hour first thing in the morning and felt particularly strong. Then, an hour later you felt totally exhausted. Write it down. This may help you realize that you skipped breakfast that morning, or perhaps you over trained the day before. I also recommend recording what you eat throughout the day. Start today! Grab your phone and download a fitness-tracking app (see Resources page 122), or if you are like me, pick up your notebook. It can be surprisingly therapeutic to work toward your goals on paper. Start by logging your current weight and measurements. (I've included a section of notebook pages in the back of this book if you'd like to get started.)

HOW OFTEN SHOULD I WEIGH MYSELF?

Here is a better question: How often do you feel like throwing the scale out the window? I can totally identify. It is amazing to me how an inanimate object like a scale can have so much power. Understand that the scale is a poor indicator of whether or not you are in shape. Your body composition is not simply determined by how much you weigh, but by how much of your body weight comes from fat. Appropriate amounts of both fat and lean tissue are necessary for optimal health. The average body fat percentage for a healthy woman is 20 to 25 percent.

A popular way to measure body fat is with a skin-fold caliper. A trainer will pinch certain sites on your body to get a measurement. It is not completely accurate, but it does give you a good picture. Also, did you know that your weight can fluctuate throughout the day? And we are not talking about the pound that comes off when you take off your shoes to weigh yourself. It's normal for a person's weight to change a few pounds from day to day. For one thing, what you're eating can make a dramatic short-term difference. Foods that are high in sodium can cause water retention, which is often the culprit when a few unexpected pounds register on the scale. Often, weighing ourselves becomes a compulsion, a "weigh" of seeing if we are worthy of reward. If you are serious about dieting, don't play mind games with yourself. I recommend weighing in no more than once a week, and I strongly discourage weighing yourself every day! If you're exercising regularly and keeping your diet in check, your weight shouldn't fluctuate enough to cause you concern.

Your "dream weight" is just that—a dream. One of the worst things you can do is pin your success or failure on a numerical goal that may or may not be physically attainable. And don't believe those nickel scales you see in pharmacies. There really is no "correct" weight for a certain height. How much you weigh may depend on your build, your body fat percentage, how active you are, your diet, and many other factors. You can, however, determine your body mass index (BMI), which is a handy way to keep track of your height-to-weight ratio. The easiest way to determine your body mass index, or BMI, is with this formula:

Multiply your weight (in pounds) by 704.5.
Multiply your height (in inches) by your height (in inches).
  Divide the first result by the second.
Example: A 5-foot 2-inch, 120-pound woman
120 x 704.5 = 84,540
62 inches x 62 inches = 3,844
84,540 / 3,844 = 21.9

A BMI of 25 to 29.9 is considered overweight, and 30 or above is considered obese. More accurate measures of body fat exist—total body water, for example, or total body potassium—but they require expensive instruments that are not readily available. What's most important is that you feel good about who you are right now. Until you like yourself as is, trying to change your body shape will be a losing proposition. Self-esteem is important to maintaining a healthy, balanced lifestyle—and it's a definite must if successful weight loss is one of your goals. So it's time to smile back at that image in the mirror and value all the wonderful characteristics of the person reflected there.

TRACKING YOUR GOALS

Take two full-body pictures, front and side views, and tape them to the first pages in your notebook. Update your diary monthly with new pictures. When you are feeling discouraged, you can refer back to your previous entries to see results over time. Nothing is more motivating than seeing changes in your physique.

Here are the details you should include:
Current weight
Desired weight loss
Current measurements: Bust__ Waist__ Hips__ Thigh__ Arm__
Current dress size
Desired dress size
Overall goals
Photos

Now that we have a clear idea of what your weight loss and fitness goals are, let's do a posture assessment. First, sit up straight and read the next section.

DEVELOPING BETTER POSTURE

A radiant, attractive, confident walk down the aisle will not come from walking with a book on your head like beauty pageant contestants of the past. The muscles you engage to look graceful are used in most exercises, and keeping them limber and healthy is essential to improving your posture and preventing many common injuries. Just as you wouldn't build a house without making sure all the wood was straight, you cannot get the full benefit of a workout without maintaining proper form (posture) and improving flexibility (see Chapter 1).

Posture is not just how you carry yourself throughout the day. It's how your muscles have been conditioned to carry you. Simply, if you stand with your shoulders back, chest high, and back straight, you're on your way to good posture. If your shoulders and back are rounded and your chest is sunken, well, you guessed it . . . To improve your posture you must stretch tight muscles and strengthen weak ones.

THE FIRST STEP

Do you know where your neutral (natural, at rest) posture is? When you stand up straight, are your hands resting by your outer thighs or in front of the thigh? If those fingers fall naturally toward the front, that tells me that you may have overdeveloped, shortened pectoral (chest) and anterior deltoid (front of the shoulder) muscles. It also tells me that your hip flexors (front of hip) may be tight and your lower back may be weak. Awareness of your neutral posture can help assess and improve your own posture.

Using a yardstick as a guide, place a piece of masking tape down the center of a full-length mirror. Then place a piece of masking tape from one side of the mirror to the other at about shoulder height. If possible, add another piece around pelvic level. Make sure each line of tape is even and parallel.

Stand in front of the mirror as you would normally, placing yourself in the center, and review. If possible, have your fiancé photograph you front and side.

Are you really centered? Does your head tilt more to one side than the other? Is one hip higher than the other? Is one shoulder higher than the other? When you face sideways, does your head pitch forward? Are your shoulders in front of the vertical line?

Awareness of spinal and pelvic placement is necessary to perform not only the exercises in this book, but all exercises. When you look at your whole body in profile, the spine should have a curvature. I want to be clear. Achieving a straight spine is not your goal. You neck region curves inward, your midback curves just slightly backward, your lower back curves inward, and your tailbone curves slightly back.

Once you realize that your posture is not perfect, you can do many things to improve it. If you sit at a desk for 3 hours or more behind a computer screen or spend all day looking down at your cell phone (what I like to call "Facebook neck"), your muscles in front (chest, shoulder, abdominals) adapt to this position and become "shortened." Your posterior (back) muscles become excessively lengthened due to weak or poorly used deep muscles in the wall of your spine.

To correct this, first visualize how your spine is supposed to look. When sitting, standing, or walking, try not to slouch. We all do it. When you catch yourself slouching, take a few minutes to correct it. When you run or jog, watch your gait. Are you taking bigger steps with one leg than the other? Do you always run the same way on the same path? This may cause muscular imbalances and lead to strains and other injuries. Reverse or retrace your path so both sides of your body experience the same impact. For instance, when running on a track, do the same number of laps in each direction.

Here are a few exercises and stretches I recommend you include in your current routine:

Bent-Over *T* Raises: Stand (you can do this seated) with feet aligned beneath your hips. Bend your knees slightly and fold your upper body forward, allowing your arms to hang straight down, as pictured. Raise your arms parallel to the floor to create the letter T and lower to start position. Aim for 20 to 25 repetitions. See Wedding Dress Workouts page 59 for a step-by-step diagram.

Swimming: Lie on your stomach, completely outstretched, with the arms and legs fully extended. Reach your fingertips for the wall in front of you and your toes to the wall behind you as you simultaneously lift the right arm and left leg off the floor, as pictured. Hold them there as you lift your head and chest off the floor. Switch the arms and legs until you have a light "splashing" motion. Aim for 30 repetitions. See Wedding Dress Workouts page 35 for a step-by-step diagram.

Russian Twist: Sit on the ground with your knees bent and your heels about 2 feet from your butt. Lean slightly back, as pictured, without rounding your spine. Holding a 6-pound medicine ball, extend your arms straight out in front of you. Hands should be level with the bottom of your rib cage. Pull your navel in and twist to the left, back to center, and to the right. Aim for 30 repetitions. See Wedding Dress Workouts page 47 for a step-by-step diagram.

Hamstring Stretch: Lie down on your back and flex hip and knee to a 90-degree angle, as pictured. Keep your low back flat on the floor as you slowly extend the knee to the ceiling. Hold the stretch for at least 20 to 30 seconds. See Wedding Dress Workouts page 43.

Chest Stretch: Stand straight with knees bent. Extend arms behind your back and link fingers. See Wedding Dress Workouts page 31. Hold the stretch for at least 20 to 30 seconds.

It's simple: Improve your physical carriage and bolster your overall health and fitness. The irony is that people associate good posture with stiffness, but nothing could be further from the truth. Flexibility, maximized by regular stretching, is the foundation of proper posture. Besides the obvious benefit to your back and neck, good posture is also a mood enhancer. Looking good means feeling great. Take the time to improve your posture. As you take the stroll down the aisle, everyone around you will "sit up" and take notice.

CHAPTER 3

Wedding Dress Workouts

ow that you have selected the perfect dress, it's time to focus on the assets that your particular dress will show off. Find the dress style that most closely matches your dress, and then incorporate the exercises I recommend for that style into your current workout routine. If your dress is a combination of different features and styles, then try more than one workout.

Before you start, make sure you select weights that are challenging. No, you are *not* going to get bulky using weights. That's a myth that just keeps women from getting strong. When you're training efficiently, your last repetitions should feel really hard and you should not be able to do another without compromising proper form. But remember the basics from Chapter 1; the following exercises are only part of the battle. You must incorporate a healthy-eating plan (which you'll find in Chapter 6) and a regular cardio program (see Chapter 5).

THE SWEETHEART NECKLINE

If your dress is plunging in the front or back, make sure it looks great! Sweetheart necklines require your "bust to rise to the occasion" while open backs are asking you to "bring sexy back." Tone the muscles of the chest and back with the following exercises.

Do these four exercises in a circuit. Repeat 2 to 3 times.

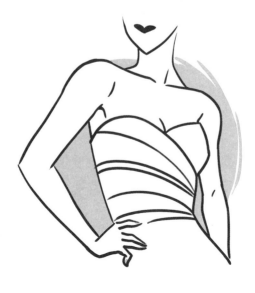

While it won't increase your cup size, a few push-ups each day will help lift and define your chest, giving a fuller, shapelier appearance. Love 'em? Hate 'em? Just do them! Push-ups are by far my favorite upper-body exercise. In fact, if I had to choose only one exercise to do for my upper body for the rest of my life, nothing beats the push-up. It always shows me my fitness level. If it feels too difficult to do, it means one of two things: I've been slacking off and letting myself get weak, or I'm packing on the pounds. Either way, it is time for me to work harder and watch my diet! Not only are push-ups the best, they are something almost everybody can do. Barring spinal injuries and rotator cuff issues, and unless you've specifically been told not to do push-ups by your doctor or medical practitioner, you should do them.

Here's a bunch of fun (okay, maybe not so fun!) ways to do a push-up, from easiest to hardest.

First, select your level:

The beginner push-up, also known as a "girl push-up," begins on hands and knees, as pictured, with your hands slightly wider than shoulder-width apart and the pelvis shifted forward.

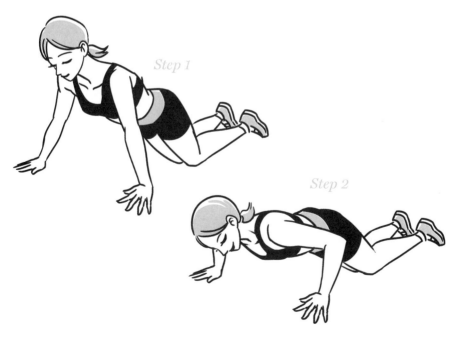

Step 1

Step 2

The standard push-up begins on hands and feet. Keep your hands slightly wider than shoulder-width apart, with fingers spread and pointing straight ahead. For both versions, keep your back straight, your abs contracted, your booty down, and your spine aligned. The start or "up" position is with your arms straight. Inhale as you lower yourself toward the floor and exhale as you push yourself up from the floor. Aim for 15 to 20 repetitions.

Once you master the basic push-up, challenge yourself with a variety of hand positions. Add a stability ball or incorporate other exercise, like push-up to side plank, push-up with a mountain climb, squat thrust to a push-up, or push-up to a one-arm row. If you need more instructions or ideas, e-mail me at BonneMarcus@gmail.com.

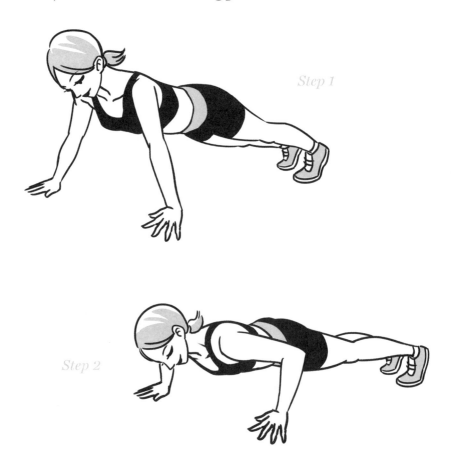

Step 1

Step 2

Push-up With Stability Ball

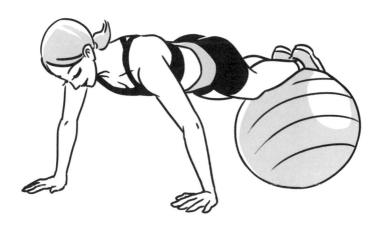

Push-up With Medicine Ball

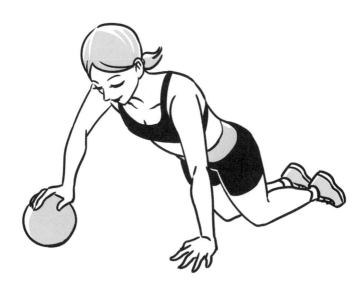

Incline Chest Press

Select a pair of 10- to 12-pound dumbbells and sit on the floor with a stability ball between your back and a wall. With your upper back resting against the ball, lift the dumbbells, palms forward, wrists straight, to shoulder height, with your arms at a 90 degree angle. Slowly raise your arms up until your elbows are straight but not locked, maintaining a straight wrist, then slowly lower to the start position to complete one repetition. Aim for 20 repetitions.

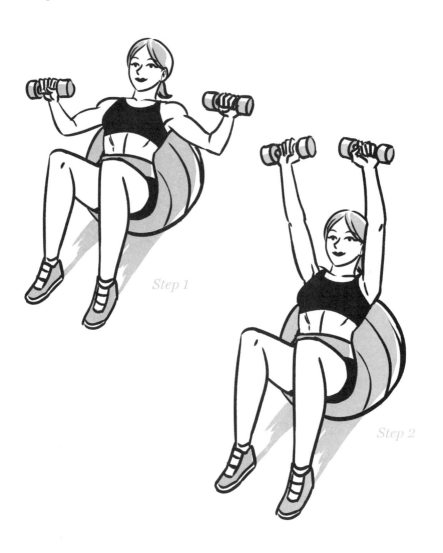

Step 1

Step 2

Stability Ball Chest Fly

Select a pair of 8- to 10-pound dumbbells and sit upright on a stability ball, resting the dumbbells on your knees. Slowly lie back on the ball, simultaneously rolling forward so that your back and head are on the ball, your knees bent, as in Step 1. Raise your arms over your chest. Your arms should be straight, but don't lock your elbows, and remember to keep your wrists straight throughout. Bring the dumbbells directly over your chest, palms facing, arms shoulder width apart. Slowly lower your arms out, maintaining a slight bend at the elbow, and stopping when the dumbells are even with your shoulder. Don't hyper-extend past that point. Slowly lift the dumbbells to return to the start position to complete one repetition. Aim for 20 repetitions.

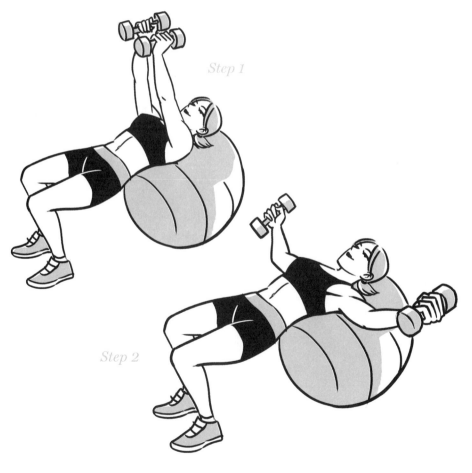

Step 1

Step 2

Wrap the band around a sturdy object like a banister behind you at chest level. Take the handles and fully extend the arms (avoid locking out the elbows) with the palms facing in, as pictured. Open the arms out to the side until they are in line with your shoulders and squeeze the chest as you bring your arms together. Aim for 25 to 30 repetitions.

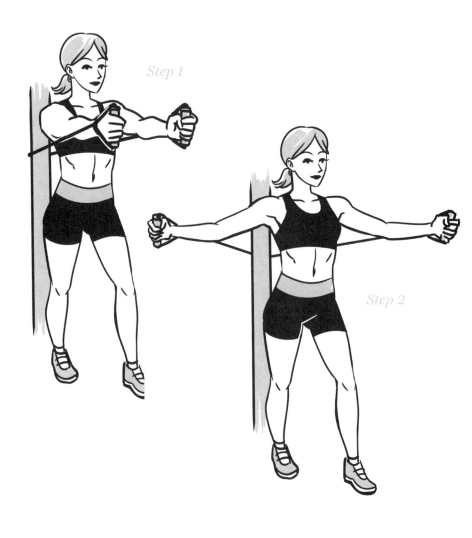

Step 1

Step 2

DON'T FORGET TO STRETCH!

Stand straight with your knees bent. Extend your arms behind your back and link fingers—hold the stretch for at least 20 to 30 seconds.

While push-ups, presses, and flys offer effective ways to lift your breasts, there is one foolproof way to give rise to the bustline. Mom was right when she lectured you about your posture—whether you're an A-cup or a D-cup, stand up straight! When you stand with your back straight and your shoulders back, you give "the girls" a lift and look great.

Another way to improve your posture, prevent a hunched look, and give rise to the bustline is to strengthen the muscles of the upper back and shoulders. These exercises are also perfect for those open-back wedding gowns.

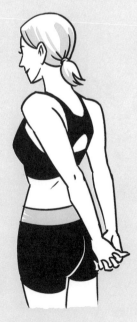

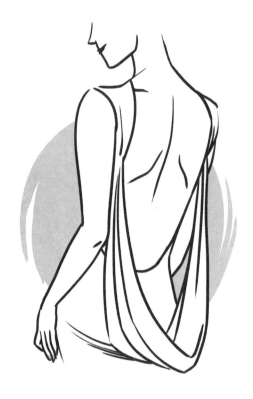

THE OPEN-BACK DRESS

If you are one of the many brides-to-be preparing to walk down the aisle in an open-back or halter-top gown, but the view from the back is less than desirable, here are a few of my favorite upper-back and shoulder exercises that will enhance your posture.

Do the following three exercises in a circuit. Repeat 2 to 3 times.

Vertical Row with the Equalizer

This inverted row is great for the upper back and biceps muscles. To do this right, make sure the Equalizer bars are set up as shown. Keep your head in a neutral position, your hips up, and your feet flat on the floor with knees bent, as pictured. Pull up as high as possible, pause for a count of 2, and lower slowly. Aim for 15 to 20 repetitions.

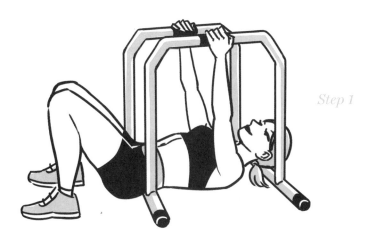

Step 1

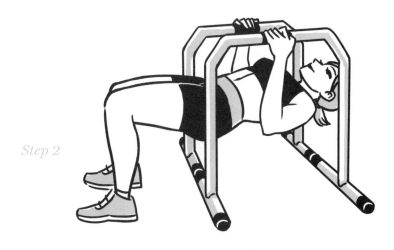

Step 2

Wrap the band around a stationary object at about waist height. When you're seated, the band should be in line with your chest. Sit on the stability ball, holding the band, as pictured, remembering to keep your elbows soft. (You can do this exercise standing as well.) Pull the arms back, slightly grazing your sides as you pull your elbows behind your rib cage. As you draw your arms back, squeeze your shoulder blades together and slowly return to start, and repeat. Aim for 25 to 30 repetitions.

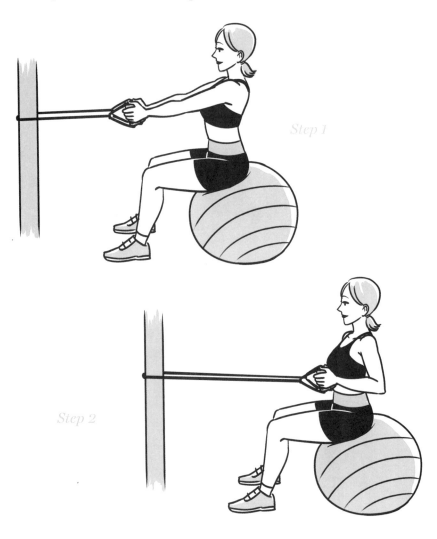

Step 1

Step 2

Swimming

Lie on your stomach, completely outstretched, with the arms and legs fully extended. Reach your fingertips for the wall in front of you and your toes to the wall behind you as you simultaneously lift the right arm and left leg off the floor, as pictured. Hold them there as you lift your head and chest off the floor. Switch the arms and legs until you have a light "splashing" motion. Aim for 30 repetitions.

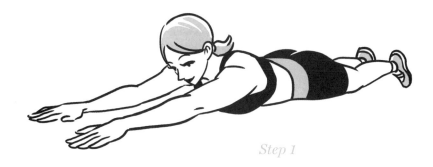

Step 1

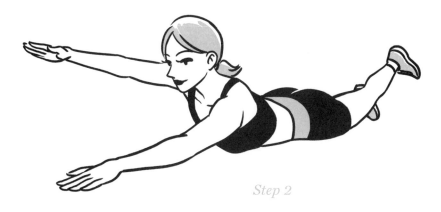

Step 2

Position yourself, as pictured, with both your arms extended in front of you, your hands clasped together. Round your mid and upper back and drop your chin to your chest as you reach forward with both of your arms. Hold the stretch for at least 20 to 30 seconds.

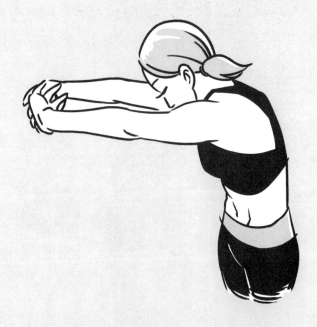

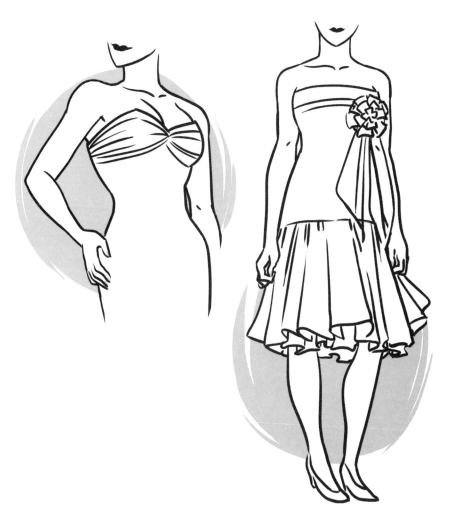

THE FORM-FITTED GOWN

Get an *abs*olutely great view from the front or the back! Form-fitted and sheath dresses cling to the body, drawing attention to the booty, abs, and thighs. And let's not forget about short wedding gowns that show off those gorgeous legs of yours.

Do the following five exercises in a circuit. Repeat 2 to 3 times.

Standing with good posture, place the gliding disc under the ball of your left foot, as pictured. Keep your left leg straight as you fully glide your leg back until you can reach the floor with your left hand. Allow the body to bend forward so there is a straight line running from the crown of your head to your heel. Your right knee bends, but make sure it does not go past your toes. Pulling against the resistance of the disc, glide your left leg back up to a standing position. Aim for 25 repetitions per leg.

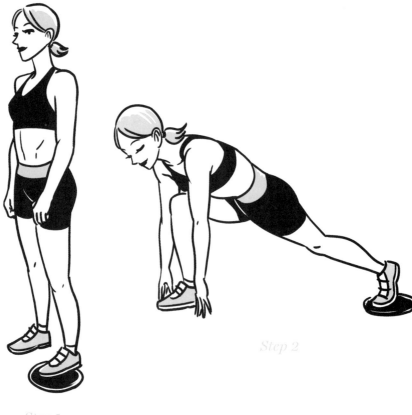

Step 1

Step 2

Hold a 6-pound medicine ball in front of your chest, as pictured. Begin the lunge by taking a large step. Lower your hips and allow your right knee to drop to a point just before it touches the floor. Hold the lunge position and rotate the upper body to the left and back to center. Step the left foot back to meet the right and repeat on the opposite leg. Aim for 25 repetitions per leg.

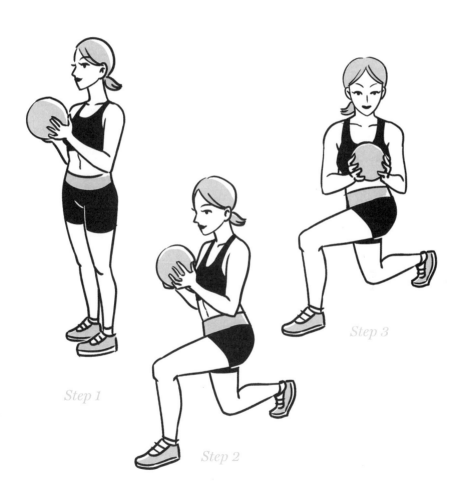

Step 1

Step 2

Step 3

Plié Squat with a Side Bend

Stand with your feet together, your toes and knees turned out comfortably, holding a medicine ball as pictured. Keep your back straight and abs contracted. As you take a big step to the right, bend your knees and lower your hips (think of yourself sliding down an imaginary wall) into a squat and raise the ball above your head. Holding the squat position, bend to the right and return to center before dragging your right foot to the start position. Do all 25 repetitions on the right side and repeat on the other side.

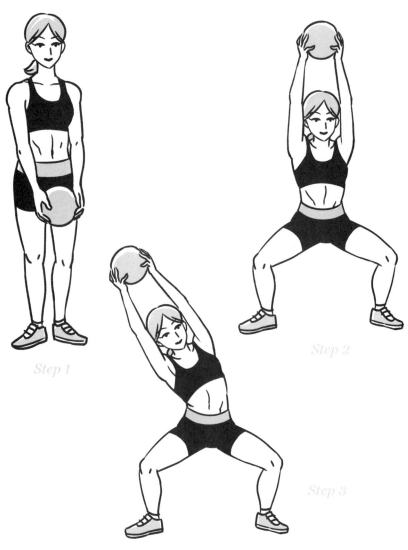

Step 1

Step 2

Step 3

Single Leg Hip Extension

Lie on your back with one foot on the stability ball and raise one foot into the air, as pictured. Push the hips up until your hips are at full extension. Return to the starting position and repeat with the other leg. Aim for 25 repetitions per leg.

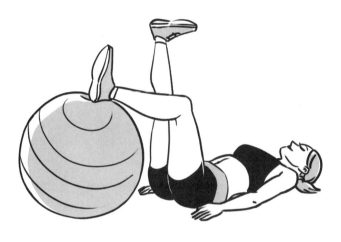

Step 1

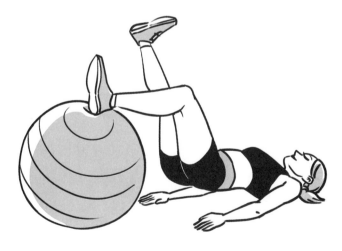

Step 2

Bridge with Plié

Lie on the floor with the legs straight and feet turned out slightly on a stability ball, as pictured. Lift and hold the glutes off the floor as you roll the ball toward you and return to the start position. Aim for 25 repetitions.

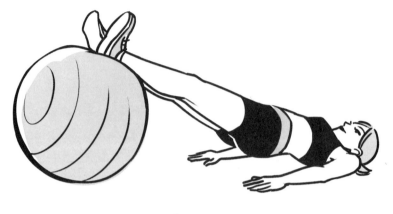

Step 1

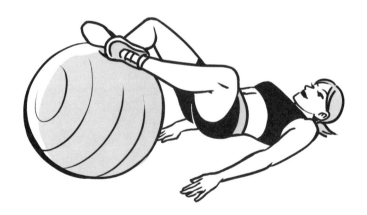

Step 2

DON'T FORGET TO STRETCH!

HAMSTRINGS: Lie down on your back and flex your hips and knees to a 90-degree angle, as pictured. Keep your lower back flat on the floor as you slowly straighten your leg to the ceiling. Hold the stretch for at least 20 to 30 seconds.

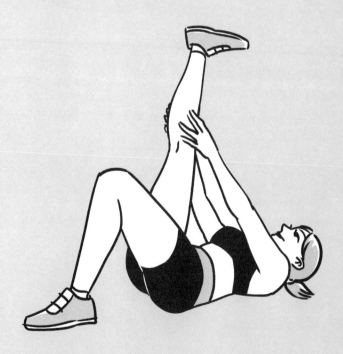

HIPS AND GLUTES: Sit with good posture, as pictured, creating a triangle with your legs by placing your right foot on top of your left knee and right knee on top of your left foot, and hinge slightly forward until the stretch is felt. Hold the stretch for at least 20 to 30 seconds. Return to the upright position, cross your legs in the opposite direction, and repeat.

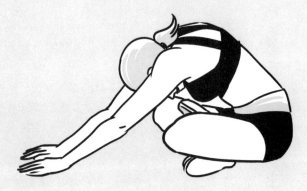

QUADRICEPS: Stand with good posture and grasp one ankle, as pictured. Keep your knees parallel to each other and tip your tailbone under slightly. Hold the stretch for at least 20 to 30 seconds. Switch sides.

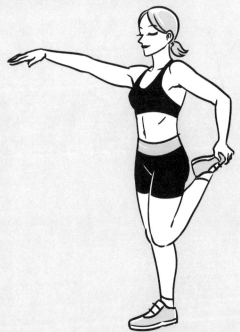

To strengthen your core, do the following four exercises in a circuit. Repeat 2 to 3 times.

Gliding Disc Tucks

Get into the plank position with your hands on the floor and both feet on top of a gliding disc, as pictured. Bring your knees in toward your chest and then extend your legs back to the starting position. Make sure that you keep your hands directly underneath your shoulders and keep your core muscles engaged as you extend your legs so that your back does not arch. Aim for 30 repetitions.

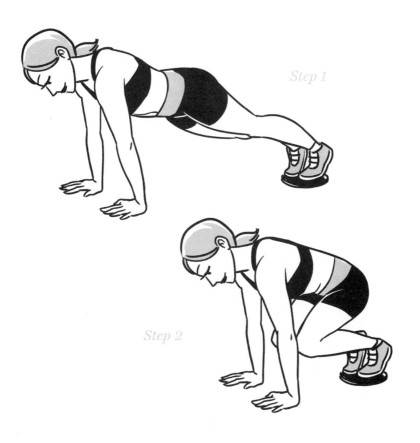

Step 1

Step 2

Lay with your middle back on the stability ball, feet shoulder-width apart, with your hands behind your head, as pictured. Keep your chin off your chest and slowly curl forward, bringing your rib cage toward your hips. Slowly return to start position and repeat 30 times. Add a twist to target the waistline. Aim for 30 repetitions side to side.

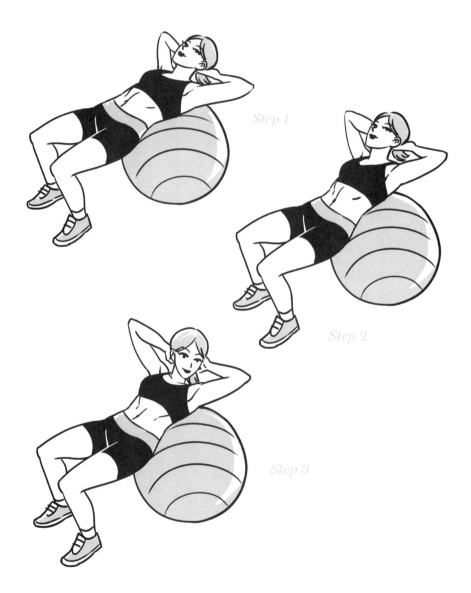

Step 1

Step 2

Step 3

Bicycles

Lie on your back, keeping your lower back pressed into the floor and flattening the arch of your lower back. Place your fingers on the side of your head just behind your ears. Bend your knees so that your thighs are at about a 90-degree angle to the floor. Simultaneously lift your shoulders off the floor and bring your right elbow to your left knee while extending the right leg, as pictured. Use a slow bicycle-pedaling motion as you switch sides. Aim for 40 to 50 repetitions.

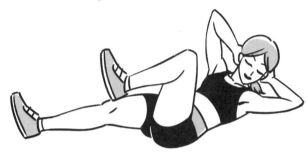

Russian Twist

Sit on the ground with your knees bent and your heels about 2 feet from your butt. Lean slightly back, as pictured, without rounding your spine. Holding a 6-pound medicine ball, extend your arms straight out in front of you. Hands should be level with the bottom of your rib cage. Pull your navel in and twist to the left, then back to center, and then rotate to the right. Aim for 30 repetitions.

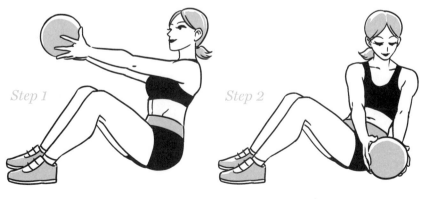

Step 1 *Step 2*

COBRA: Lie on your stomach. Place your hands by the side of your body, in line with your chest, as pictured. Push your pelvis and hips into the floor as you lift your chest off the floor. Hold the stretch for at least 20 to 30 seconds.

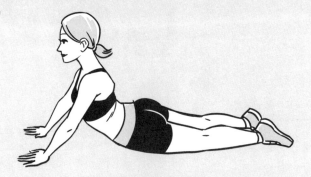

CROSS LEG ROTATION: Lie down on your back with your knees bent at a 90-degree angle. Cross the right leg over the left and rotate the lower body to the left while keeping both shoulder blades and palms in contact with the floor, as pictured. Hold the stretch for at least 20 to 30 seconds. Switch sides and repeat.

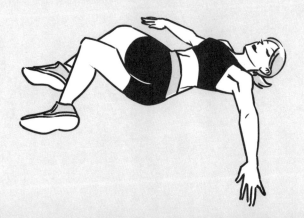

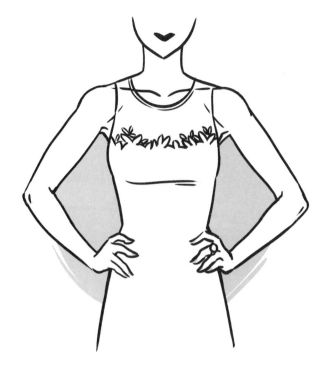

THE SLEEVELESS GOWN

Armed for the *big day*! If you are one of the many brides-to-be preparing to walk down the aisle in a halter, tank top, spaghetti strap, or strapless gown but your ar ms and shoulders aren't looking anything like you'd really like them to look, here are a few of my favorite arm and shoulder exercises to help you tone your arms for the big day.

Do the following six arm exercises in a circuit. Repeat 2 to 3 times.

Kneel approximately an arm's length away from the bar, as pictured, and position your hands shoulder-width apart. Maintain alignment from the shoulder to the knee and slowly lower your body toward the Equalizer bar by dropping the elbows. Return to the start position by straightening the arms. Aim for 20 repetitions.

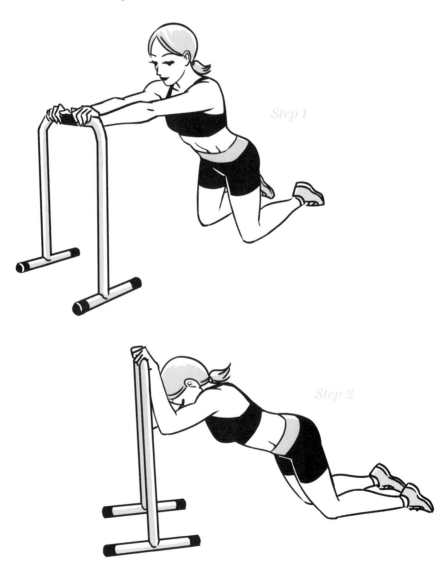

Step 1

Step 2

Body Bar Biceps Curls

Stand with good posture, holding a Body Bar with the arms shoulder width apart, palms facing up as pictured. Curl the arms up to the shoulders and lower slowly. Keep your wrists straight, don't let them roll toward you as you raise the bar. Aim for 15 to 20 repetitions.

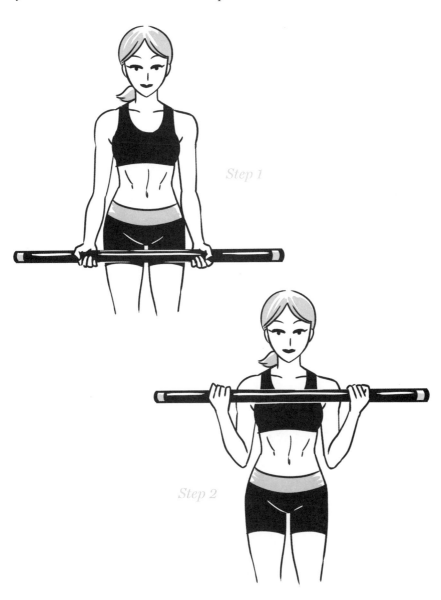

Step 1

Step 2

Position yourself on your knees with a resistance band under your shins, as pictured. Hold the band in both hands and raise your arms above your head, biceps aligned next to your ears. Bend your elbows to a 90-degree angle behind your head and then fully extend the arms without locking your elbows. Aim for 20 to 25 repetitions.

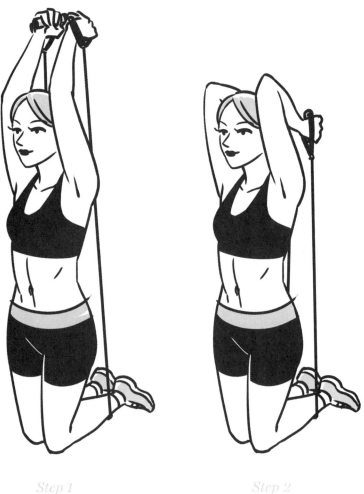

Step 1   *Step 2*

Biceps Curl with a Resistance Band

Wrap the band around your feet, as pictured. With your arms extended, palms facing up, holding the band as pictured, curl both arms toward your shoulders. Keep your wrists straight, don't let them roll toward you as you raise the band. Aim for 20 to 25 repetitions.

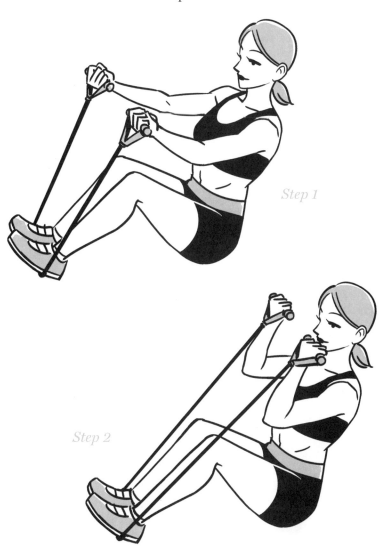

Step 1

Step 2

Lie down on your back with your knees bent. Holding 8- to 10-pound dumbbells, extend your arms as pictured, and keeping your wrists straight throughout the exercise. Bring the right elbow to the floor, and as you extend the right arm up, simultaneously lower the left elbow to the floor. Aim for 20 to 25 repetitions. On the last repetition, extend both arms to the start position. Then bend both arms at the elbow, bringing the weights close to the floor on opposite sides of your head, next to your ears. Straighten the arms, making sure to keep the upper arm and elbow stationary throughout the movement. Aim for 20 to 25 repetitions.

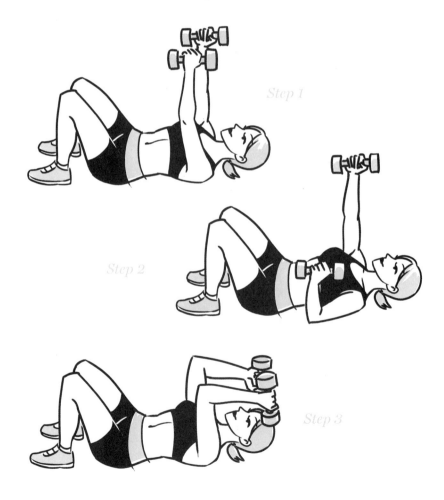

Standing with knees slightly bent hold a pair of 8- to 10-pound dumbbells. Position one arm at a 90-degree angle and the other arm straight, as pictured. While one arm curls the dumbbell, the other arm remains in a static hold. Do 5 repetitions per am and switch arms 4 times.

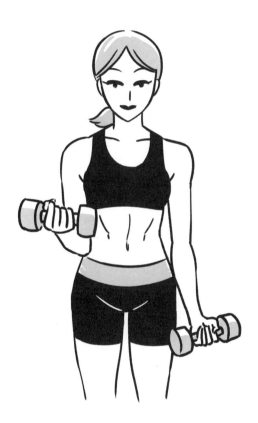

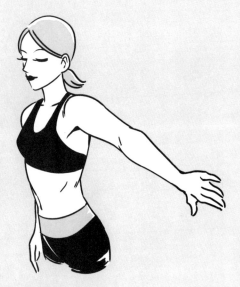

BICEPS: As pictured, extend the arm out to the side with the thumb down and palm facing back. Hold the stretch for at least 20 to 30 seconds. Repeat with other arm.

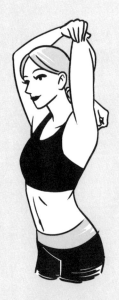

TRICEPS: As pictured, reach up and over with one arm, assisting with the other. Hold the stretch for at least 20 to 30 seconds. Switch sides.

More Exercises for Sexy Shoulders
Do the following three exercises in a circuit. Repeat 2 to 3 times.

Alternating L Raises

Stand with your right arm by your side and your left arm in front of your thigh, as pictured. Raise both arms to create the letter *L*, lower to start position, switch arms, and repeat. Aim for 20 to 25 repetitions.

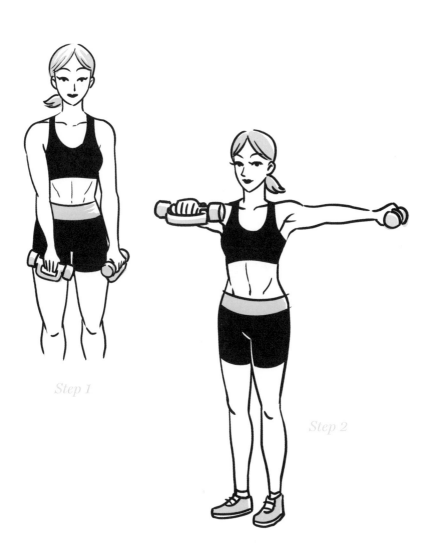

Step 1

Step 2

V Press

Hold weights just above your shoulders, as pictured. Press your arms up and out slightly so that at the top of the motion your arms create the letter *V.* Aim for 20 to 25 repetitions.

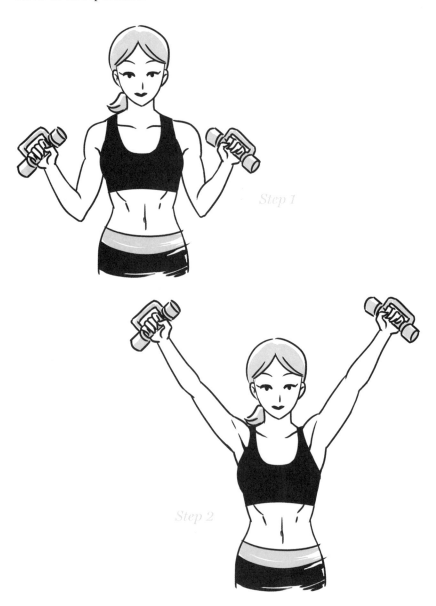

Step 1

Step 2

Stand (or, alternatively, sit) with feet aligned beneath your hips. Bend your knees slightly and fold your upper body forward, allowing your arms to hang straight down, as pictured. Raise your arms parallel to the floor to create the letter *T* and lower to start position. Aim for 20 to 25 repetitions.

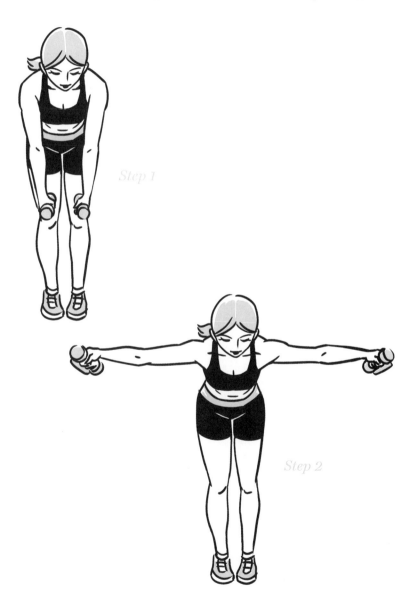

Step 1

Step 2

SHOULDERS: As pictured, reach one arm across the body, assisting with the other.

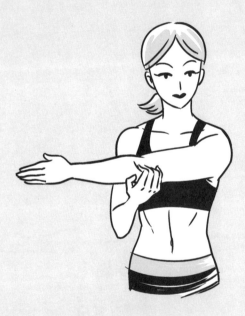

While the workout moves in this chapter target your gown-specific goals, there is one caveat: Don't focus *only* on the one or two body parts you'd like to improve. Focus on conditioning your *entire* body, which will lower your total body fat and increase overall lean muscle mass.

Before you know it, you will tighten, tone, and transform yourself into that fairy-tale princess bride.

CHAPTER 4

The Ultimate Down-the-Aisle Workout

Your walk down the aisle is a moment fixed in time. It is an experience that can never be duplicated—so you'll want to look and feel amazing. When those doors open, your loving groom will be waiting for you at the end of the aisle. I mean, come on: perfect man, perfect gown, perfect day, perfect you. It's your wedding day and you want to look better than you have looked . . . *ever!*

My ultimate Down-the-Aisle workout will help you release that radiant and confident woman that can't wait to walk down the aisle and into the next chapter of her life. Designed to blast fat and burn calories fast, this targeted program combines quick, agility-based cardio drills with innovative strength-training exercises that work together to boost your metabolism, burn calories, and reshape your body. Effective and intense, it will clean out the cobwebs of your previous exercise routines to increase your energy and your mood.

All the exercises, including warm-up and cardio, are done while moving "down an aisle." Freestanding exercises like plié squats and lunges are effective. But when you perform these same exercises with movement across a floor, you kick up the intensity, engage more muscles, and improve balance. The addition of upper-body movements with light or moderate weights provides an extra layer of muscle strengthening. Another bonus is that by integrating these movements, you train your core. In other words, you get more bang for your buck—for your abs as well as your butt!

The Down-the-Aisle workout has a warm-up, five strength-based exercises, and five cardio drills. The workout requires a medicine ball and a set of 3- to 8-pound dumbbells. The strength-based exercises can be done in a bedroom as 1 repetition from side to side. The workout is designed for an area of approximately 20 to 30 yards (about the length of a gym floor) or approximately 25 repetitions on each leg.

A few ground rules:

Always warm up first. Do an easy jog up and down the "aisle"
for 5 minutes.
Follow each strength move with a burst of cardio: Do 90
seconds to 2 minutes of cardio to get your heart pumping
in between each strength move.

The ultimate Down-the-Aisle workout will increase energy, burn fat, and build muscle.

Walking Lunges with a Triceps Extension into a Wood Chop

(Great for your glutes, legs, arms, and abs)

Stand with good posture: shoulders back and abdominals contracted. Hold a 6-pound medicine ball behind your head, as pictured. As you take a large step forward (heel then toe of the left foot), lower your body until the left thigh is parallel to the floor, and extend the arms forward and over, bringing the medicine ball to the outside of the front left thigh. You allow your trailing right knee to drop to a point just before it touches the floor. Swing the medicine ball up and over your head as you bring your feet together. As you move across the floor or down your hallway, step forward with the right leg.

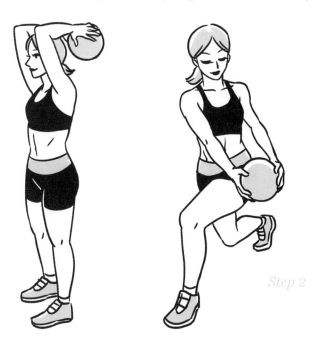

Step 1

Step 2

Jog forward, turn around, and jog back. Move quickly, as if you were chasing your fiancé. Aim for 90 seconds to 2 minutes.

Inchworm Push-Ups

(Great for your legs, chest, arms, and abs)

From a standing position, with your feet together or slightly apart, engage ("brace") your abdominal muscles to stabilize your spine. Gently exhale and bend forward from your hips ("hip hinging"). Try to keep your knees straight (but not locked). Slowly lower your torso toward the floor until you

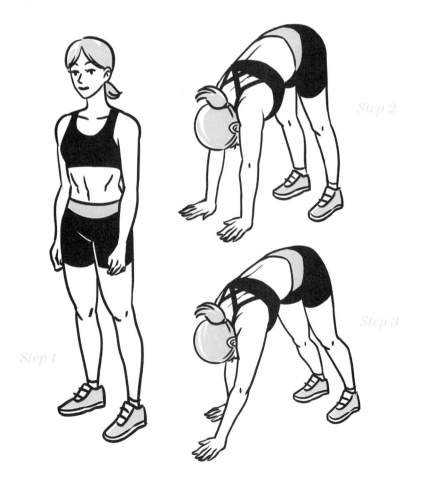

Step 1

Step 2

Step 3

can place your fingers or palms on the floor in front of your body. If your hamstrings are tight, you may need to bend your knees slightly. Slowly begin to walk your hands forward, away from your feet. Your heels will begin to rise off the floor. Continue walking your hands forward until you reach a full push-up position, where your spine, hips, and head are level with the floor (plank position). Perform one full push-up, bending the elbows and lowering your chest and hips simultaneously to the floor. Press up to plank position, keeping the abs engaged and your head aligned with your spine. Slowly begin walking your feet forward toward your hands, taking steps without moving your hands. Maintain a flat spine throughout and continue walking until your feet are close to your hands. Repeat this movement and continue down the aisle.

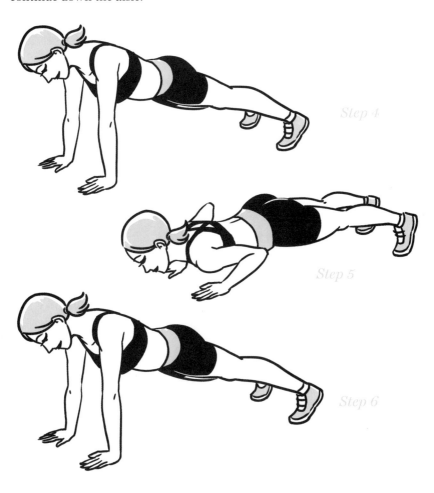

Step 4

Step 5

Step 6

Side Shuffles

Quickly shuffle your right leg out to your side, followed by your left leg, bringing them together, and repeat (like galloping when you were a kid). Aim for 90 seconds to 2 minutes.

Plié Squat Travel with a Front Raise and Twist

(Great for your glutes, inner thighs, shoulders, and abs)
Stand with your feet together, your toes and knees turned out, comfortably holding a 6-pound medicine ball, as pictured. Keep your back straight and

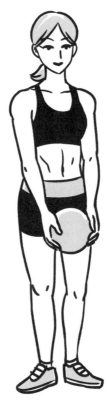

Step 1

abs contracted. As you take a big step to the right, bend your knees and lower your hips (think of sliding down an imaginary wall) into a squat. Raise the ball to shoulder level. Holding the squat position, twist your torso to the right just beyond your right knee. Return to center before dragging your left foot to the right. Reverse the direction by taking a big step with the left foot.

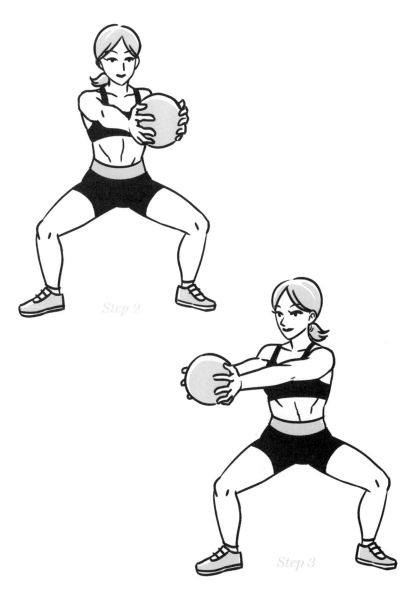

Step 2

Step 3

Lateral Hops and Backpedal (Jog Backward)

Begin with both feet together and push off to the side with one leg moving forward on a diagonal, followed by the other foot creating a zigzag formation. Upon landing, immediately push off in the opposite direction to end and then backpedal (jog) to the opposite end. Repeat this pattern for 90 seconds to 2 minutes.

Squat with Hammer Curl

(Great for your glutes, thighs, and arms)
Stand up straight with dumbbells in front of your shoulders, as pictured. Step out to the right, and as you lower down into a squat position, reaching your hips back as if you were about to sit in a chair, extend the arms straight down, as pictured. Keep most of your weight back on your heels and be careful not to extend the knees beyond the toes. Press into the heels and stand back up straight without locking the knees. As you step the left foot toward the right foot, curl the arms up.

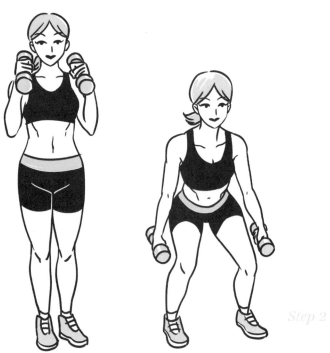

Step 1   Step 2

(Great for your glutes, arms, shoulders, and abs)

People usually crawl on their hands and knees facedown, so it may feel unnatural to be on your hands and feet face up. Sit with your legs spread out in front of you, shoulders width apart, and feet flat on the ground. Bring your arms behind you with your palms flat and gently raise yourself off the ground, tightening your gluteus muscles. Hold this position and take one step (crawl) forward, starting with your right hand and left foot, followed by your left hand and right foot. Hold this position and tap the right foot with the left hand and then the left foot with the right hand, as pictured, and continue down the aisle.

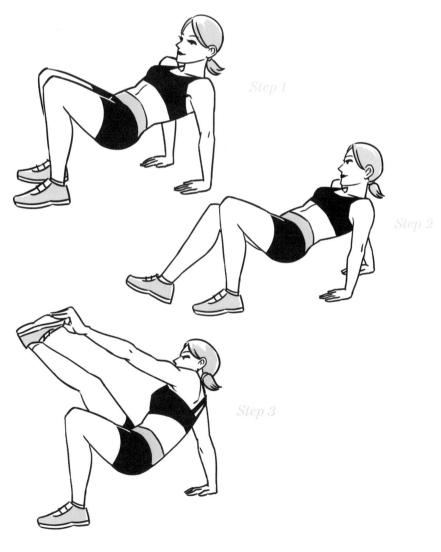

Step 1

Step 2

Step 3

Suicide Drill

This simple drill has a high cardio impact. Pick a starting point and place one object about 20 yards away from you (or approximately ⅓ the length of the gym floor) and a second object about 50 yards away from you (or approximately ⅔ the length of the gym floor). Then sprint to the first object and back to the starting position. Sprint to the second object and back to the start. Finally, sprint the entire length and back to the start. Repeat this sequence as many times as you can. Aim for 90 seconds to 2 minutes.

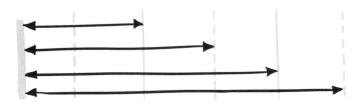

High Knee Skips/Butt Kicks Jog

Skip forward with exaggerated arms and legs to the end of the aisle. On the return, jog forward while kicking your heels to your booty. Follow this pattern for 90 seconds to 2 minutes.

A FEW MORE GROUND RULES:
- Complete the entire circuit of moves 2 or 3 times.
- Make sure you stretch after each workout.
- Stay hydrated.
- For optimum results, do this routine at least 3 times per week.
- This workout will produce results fast! Not only will you burn fat, torch calories, and build muscle, but you will unleash the diva bride who can't wait to walk down the aisle and into the next chapter of her life.

CHAPTER 5

Bridal Burn: Wedding Cardio

t's no surprise that cardiovascular exercise is the cornerstone of most weight-loss programs and the key to shedding excess body fat. Aerobic activity also nourishes a positive mental attitude by increasing the body's level of serotonin, one of the feel-good hormones that helps reduce stress (and it even comes without a doctor's prescription). And who wouldn't have stress? I mean, you are planning a wedding!

Before we continue, you must understand that you can't target exactly where you'll lose the inches. No one gets to decide where the fat burns off first. You may unhappily drop a cup size before you lose the pouch or saddlebags. I can't tell you how often I am asked why this "injustice" occurs. Mother Nature is a cruel mistress. Who knows? What we do know is fat is lost throughout the body in a pattern dependent on genetics, sex (hormones), and age. Overall body fat must be reduced in order to lose fat in any particular area. Although fat is lost or gained throughout the body, it seems the first area to get fat is generally the last area to become lean—sort of a "first hired, last fired" principle. While a little discouraging, it is also true that hard work, done correctly and thoughtfully, will yield results again and again. It can be done!

CARDIO CHOICES

So the question becomes, "What is the best cardio exercise?" The best cardio, in my opinion, is anything you will do consistently. Sure, there are arguments about whether the elliptical is better than the treadmill, or the StairMaster better than the stationary bike, but the reality is that you will reap the most benefits from any cardio that you do as long as you actually do it. The secret to success is to find an activity you love. I'm pretty fickle and share my love among running, Spinning, and jumping rope. What is the best form of cardio for you? Before you decide, check out my thoughts on the choices.

Love them! Why? In a half hour or less, depending on the intensity level, you can experience a full cardiovascular workout with little or no impact on the joints. What makes it even more appealing is the combined upper- and lower-body workout. You have a variety of workouts to choose from, and no other piece of equipment delivers a more efficient and time-saving workout. With an elliptical, you get a workout that targets the quads, hamstrings, glutes, chest, back, triceps, and biceps. The more muscles you use, the greater the energy expenditure, so you end up burning more calories and fat in less time.

Elliptical machines offer a range of workouts programmed into the machine, and require little skill. You simply put your feet on the foot pedals and begin pedaling, as your hands hold on to the moving handlebars. When you stop pedaling, the machine stops, too. The foot pedals can be worked in a forward or reverse direction. When you change the direction of the pedals, you target your lower body in different ways. Need more convincing? Then try the variety of preprogrammed workouts. They range from fat-burning and cross-country skiing to hill-climbing and target training zone programs. In the past I used the manual setting (which is *awesome* for interval training; more on that later), but once I discovered the fat-burning and hill-climbing programs, there was no going back. For each of the programs, the machine adjusts the incline and the resistance at various intervals. It's a great way to keep the routines fresh and energizing.

Try the following sample workout. You will have to modify the intensity (resistance) depending on the machine you use. For example, a resistance of 10 on a Life Fitness elliptical will feel different than on an Arc Trainer by Cybex. You will go forward on the elliptical and set the ramp somewhere in the middle. When in reverse, bring the ramp all the way to the top. Listening to music or watching television are great optional ways to stay motivated. Remember, you may make adjustments as needed. Always maintain an upright posture by keeping your shoulders back, chin up, back straight, and abdominals tight.

MINUTE	PACE (SPEED)	RESISTANCE	PERCEIVED EXERTION
1–5 (Warm-Up)	Moderate	Easy Does It	3
6–8	Fast/Moderate	Low/Medium	4–5
9–12	Moderate	Medium	5
13–15	Moderate	Medium/Hard	7–8
16–20 (In Reverse)	Fast	Low	8
21–25	Slow	Hard	7–8
26–30 (In Reverse)	Fast	Low	8
31–35	Slow	Hard	8–9
36–40 (In Reverse)	Fast	Low	8
41–45 (Cooldown)	Slow/Moderate	Easy Does It	3

TREADMILL

Love it! While it may seem that treadmills were invented by the same people who designed hamster wheels, what is basically walking or jogging in place is one of the best exercises you can do. Why? We walk upright by design. No formal instruction is necessary—unless you consider "put one foot in front of the other" instruction.

I'm not trying to sell the treadmill just because I love it so much. There are reasons not to use it—for example, if you have serious orthopedic concerns and have been told by your doctor not to set foot on it. Still, few machines can measure up to treadmills in terms of providing consistent health benefits. Burning calories is not the only reason treadmills appeal to so many people. Treadmills allow you to easily intensify the speed and difficulty of your workout. And many a late-blooming marathoner was born on a treadmill—including me.

It's also a great way to stay on track when the weather is uncooperative. Get in the car (Drive carefully. It is raining out.), head to the gym, get on your favorite treadmill, and continue with your usual outdoor pace. Even a certified couch potato can get a good workout without giving up the remote.

I am often asked, "Which is better, running or walking?" so I want to address that question here. Running and walking are both fantastic exercises. There are proven health benefits for both, but it's a matter of determining what's best for you. In terms of weight loss, running wins hands down. In general, you have to walk nearly an hour to get a weight-loss benefit similar to that of a half-hour run. However, there's much less possibility for injury associated with the low-impact stride of walking.

For me, there's just something soothing about the rhythm of my breathing and my feet hitting the ground. When I'm stressed, running (or walking if you prefer) gives me a chance to think and put some distance, emotionally, between me and my stressors, as it triggers the release of endorphins—natural chemicals that ease pain and elevate mood. Endorphins are responsible for what's called the runner's high. Do keep in mind, though, that the impact of running on your joints can be more than three times your body weight—and every step is triple the impact of walking. If you decide to run, you'll have to train your body to get used to the jarring.

As the old saying goes, you've got to walk before you run, so start off slowly and gradually build running into your routine.

Try this 40-minute high-intensity boredom-buster routine:

MINUTES 1–5: Warm up at 3.0 to 3.5 mph. (For the beginner, warm up at 2.5 to 3.0 mph and modify the rest of the settings in this routine as needed.)

MINUTES 6–10: Walking at 4.0 to 4.2 mph is a great lower-body workout. This eases you into the "zone," which helps when you are having a hard time getting motivated.

MINUTES 11–15: Add an incline of 5 or 8 percent. This is just enough to give you an awareness of your booty.

MINUTES 16–20: Increase the speed on your incline to about 4.5 to 4.8 mph for a high-intensity kick-in-the-calorie burn. You should be sweating about now!

MINUTES 21–25: Keep the speed and lose the incline for a little recovery. Get ready to turn it up a notch.

MINUTES 26–30: Increase the speed to about 5.3 to 5.8 mph.

MINUTES 31–35: Push your speed to about 5.8 to 6.2 mph. The finish is just ahead and you're going for that "runner's high."

MINUTES 36–40: You are cooling down. Gradually lower the speed of your treadmill until you are at 3.0 mph. Continue walking for another 3 to 5 minutes to lower the heart rate and prevent the blood from pooling in the working muscles, which could lead to dizziness.

STATIONARY BIKES

Another personal favorite! Stationary bikes are time-tested machines that offer a great cardio, lower-body workout. They are very easy to learn to use, and for most people, the cycling motion is natural. With your own stationary bike, you can get a health-club-quality workout, burning fat and improving heart fitness even in bad weather. Two major types of stationary bikes are upright and recumbent. The upright type looks like a regular bike, while a recumbent bike reclines at an angle. Most recumbent bikes offer bucket seats and cushioned back support and may lessen strain on knees and the lower back. A great advantage of stationary bikes over other fitness equipment is that you can very easily read while cycling because you are already sitting with your hands free and not moving up and down like you would on a treadmill. Reading will combat any boredom associated with stationary biking. Compared with running, a stationary bike provides users with a thorough low-impact workout that creates less stress on joints. The biggest complaint with bicycle users is that it is a pain in the butt—literally. The numbing discomfort in the buttocks and crotch can be equal to the sometimes mind-numbing boredom associated with riding. Two words: *bike shorts*. The money you pay for the extra padding in the crotch is money well spent when you don't have to sit on a donut pad for 3 days after your first bike workout. For the boredom-busting part, Spinning classes are a nice alternative to sitting in the middle of a gym mindlessly pedaling a stationary bike.

■ *What Is Spinning?*

Spinning is a high-energy indoor cycling group exercise class that's been around since the eighties. Trainer and ultraendurance athlete Johnny Goldberg, a.k.a. Johnny G, developed the Spinning program to bring the elements of athletic training to people of all fitness levels. Spinning integrates music, camaraderie, and visualization, and it utilizes motivation and mental training techniques. It's not just a hard-core fitness program for elite athletes. It sure can be, but the truth is that Spinning was developed as an exciting athletic training program for everyone, from beginners to skilled athletes. You can burn an average of 500 calories in a 40- to 45-minute class and use muscles you didn't know existed in your body. Most gyms with a Spinning program use specially designed bikes called the Johnny G Spinner, patented by Johnny G. The Spinner is a stationary fixed-gear bike. It has a resistance knob that is controlled manually. There are no digital readouts or heart rate monitors here. In Spinning, all you have to remember is a set of five movements and three hand positions. That's it! After an introductory class, you're off to the races or a bike tour or wherever you want to be, burning a tremendous number of calories and increasing your fitness level exponentially as you go.

JUMPING ROPE

Another top choice! Jumping rope is a fantastic no-excuses way to burn calories and lose weight. It's a complete cross-training workout that combines elements of cardiovascular and endurance training with muscle strengthening. You can jump rope at your own level of intensity for any length of time almost anywhere. In fact, in only 15 to 20 minutes, you can elevate your heart rate, work up a major sweat, get an overall energy boost, and burn an average of 300 calories, depending on your height and weight. While you probably know how great jumping rope is for shaping the calves, glutes, and quads, you may not realize that constantly turning the rope will also tone your upper body.

It's probably been a while since you last picked up a jump rope—like, not since the second grade when you were singing, "B, my name is Bonne and my husband's name is Barry [actually it's Larry], we live in Baltimore [actually Long Island, NY], and we sell barbells." (Yes, okay, I was singing that.) Let's go over a few jumping basics. First, coordination doesn't always come easy, so be patient. Since jumping rope is aerobically demanding, the best way to build stamina is to use interval training, which alternates periods of work and active recovery. Active recovery means you're still doing something, but at a lower intensity. (Read more about active recovery in the section on interval training opposite.) For example, jump rope for 3 minutes and then march in place. Repeat this 4 or 5 times and before you know it, you'll have completed your workout.

OTHER CARDIO OPTIONS

If none of the options I've discussed appeal to you, do not despair. I couldn't cover everything, but there is more. Cardio kickboxing, dancing, swimming, kayaking, and rowing . . . and there is no shortage of exercise videos. Log on to www.collagevideo.com to find one that fits you perfectly.

Whatever cardiovascular exercise you choose, maximize the effectiveness of your workout by remembering preparation and reparation. Proper warm-up and stretching will ensure safe and healthy workouts. Other things to keep in mind are the guidelines from Chapter 1 on frequency, intensity and time, a.k.a. the FIT principle—how often, how hard, and how long.

MAXIMIZE THE BURN AND
BEAT THE BOREDOM

Lack of time is the number one reason clients give me for not exercising. And once they do start exercising, boredom with a lack of results is the second reason. Interval and cross-training are two great solutions for both of these common problems. Interval training involves alternating short bursts of intense activity with what is called active recovery. Active recovery is a less intense, but still active, phase. For instance, try walking for 2 minutes, then running for 30 to 60 seconds, and alternating this pattern throughout the duration of a workout. The intensity of each interval will depend on how you are feeling and what you are trying to achieve. The same is true for the length of each interval. If, for example, you have become accustomed to walking 2 miles a day in 30 minutes, try to increase the intensity of your walk and its calorie-burning potential by picking up the pace every few minutes and then returning to your usual speed. The length of each interval doesn't matter. Vary the lengths of each one if you want. It's fun to see how much more distance you can cover by doing this.

Cross-training basically means performing a variety of different forms of aerobic exercise, either within each session—for example, biking for 15 minutes and then running for 15 minutes—or day to day—like running 2 days a week, cycling 2 days a week, and swimming 1 day a week. Besides reducing boredom, cross-training helps prevent weight-loss plateaus, boosts your overall fitness level, and reduces the risk of repetitive stress injuries. One of my favorite reasons to cross-train is that you have no excuses to miss your workout. If, for example, the pool is closed, you can go for a bike ride. Or if the weather is uncooperative, you can always do a dance video at home. No matter what you choose to do for your cardio workouts, have fun with them. Go for a hike. Skate. Do something different. Break out of the same-old, same-old mentality and discover new ways to move your body.

HONEYMOON HIGH-INTENSITY INTERVAL TRAINING

Want to supercharge your endurance? (Wink, wink.) When it comes to working up a sweat and improving your stamina, my "no equipment, no excuses" cardio blaster targets the entire body, ignites calories, and gets you honeymoon-ready. This workout is made up of several intervals that include 50 seconds of intense exercise followed by 10 seconds of rest (It's not an active recovery. It's a stand still, catch your breath recovery) repeated 4 times. "Intense" doesn't adequately describe it. It's more like 50 seconds of ultraburn.

Start with a 5-minute warm-up and then perform each of the following moves in a circuit and repeat 4 times.

High Knees

Start in a standing position and begin by running in place. Get the knees up as high as you can; the thighs should be parallel to the floor at their highest point. Stay light on your feet and keep the abs contracted.

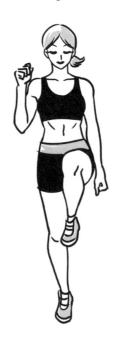

Plyo Jacks

Plyo jacks are like slow jumping jacks. You jump out, just as you would in a jumping jack, but slow things down and add a deep squat. Begin with feet together and arms by your side, as pictured. Jump the feet out, landing in a squat and circling the arms up and over the head. Jump up once again, bringing the feet together and circling the arms back down.

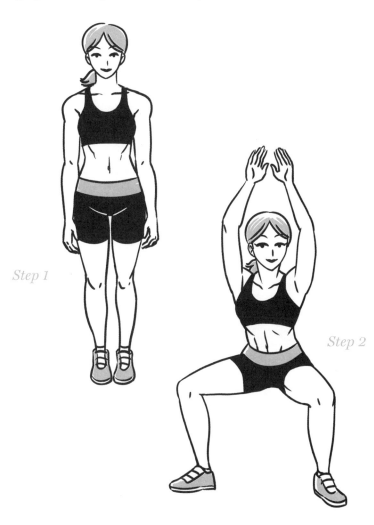

Step 1

Step 2

Bridal Burpees

Crouch down until you can rest your hands on the ground. Putting your weight on your arms, jump back and extend your legs as pictured. Your hands should be in line with your chest. Keeping the elbows tight against your torso, lower into a full push-up (see wedding dress workouts for push-ups). Push yourself up and, with another jump, bring your legs back up to your body, and then stand.

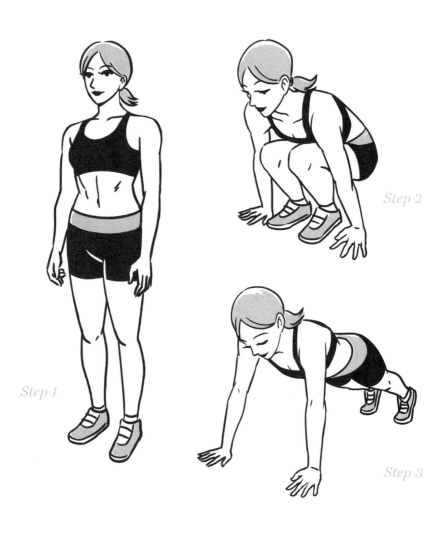

Step 2

Step 1

Step 3

Mountain Climbers

Start in a plank position, as pictured. Keep the hips in line with the shoulders as you "run the legs." Get a rhythm and stick with it.

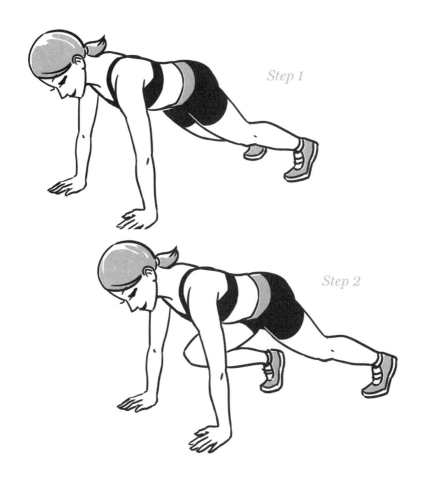

Step 1

Step 2

Tuck Jumps

Stand with feet shoulder-width apart and knees slightly bent. Bend your knees and descend to a full squat position. At the bottom of the squat, powerfully explode straight up, bringing your knees toward your chest while in midair. Grasp your knees quickly with your arms. At the top of the jump, your thighs should touch your torso. Release your legs, control your landing, and descend into the squat again for another explosive jump. Upon landing, immediately repeat the next jump.

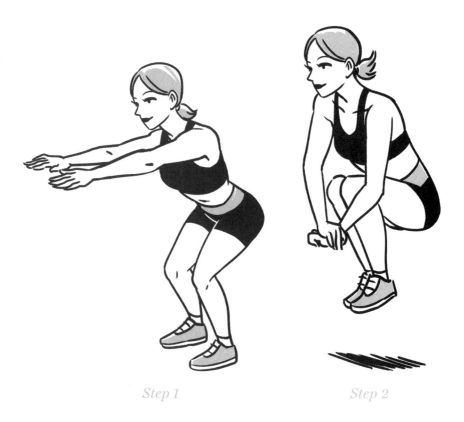

Step 1   Step 2

When it comes to cardiovascular exercise, it's worth repeating: The warm-up and cooldown are essential to the quality of the workout and your recovery. The warm-up gets you ready for work and the cooldown brings your body back to reality. Do not skip either and make sure you stretch after.

Okay, you now know all my favorite strength-training exercises and you have a great go-to workout for toning and sculpting your bridal body. However, my exercise program is incomplete without information on proper nutrition. Turn the page to learn everything you need to know.

CHAPTER 6

The Bride's Healthy-Eating Guide

ince you're making one great commitment, how about another: eating well. And by *well*, I mean healthy. Let's replace that hated word, *diet*, with a divine dining plan. Diets try to seduce you with promises of quick, drastic results, with little or no effort. Understand that all diets work in some way, but the results rarely last. Have you tried a fad diet only to be disappointed when you regain the weight? I know I have. Avoid any programs that suggest taking diet pills, eliminating any one food group, or eating unbalanced meals (like consuming only cabbage soup for a week). *Always put your health first.*

Create an eating plan that appeals to your likes but also provides the essentials. Embrace the trinity of nutrition the same way you embraced the trinity of fitness. While you can't get and stay fit without cardio, strength, and flexibility, your body needs three sisters of sustenance—protein, carbohydrate, and fat—to provide the power, energy, and harmony to function and stay healthy. In this chapter Tammy Lakatos Shames RD, LD, CDN, and her twin sister, Lyssie Lakatos, RD, LD, CDN—the "Nutrition Twins" and authors of *Fire Up Your Metabolism*—give you the "skinny" on these essential nutrients.

CARBOHYDRATES, PROTEINS, AND FATS: YOU NEED THEM ALL

Despite what you've heard, you really can't skimp on any one nutrient. Carbohydrates cannot replace the role of protein or fat; fat and protein cannot replace each other or carbohydrates.

Carbs are the last things a bride should give up as she is planning her wedding. They are your body's primary source of energy. Your brain can't run on all cylinders if you don't provide it with the fuel it needs. Imagine how difficult it would be to find the dress and wedding location of your dreams, choose the most beautiful flowers, and locate the perfect shoes and most deliciously beautiful cake without the energy carbohydrates provide.

Give up the carbs and you may not even have enough strength to make it down the aisle. Seriously, brides who avoid carbohydrates feel deprived and are prone to being grouchy and mean. *Hello, bridezilla!*

Small amounts of carbs must be part of every meal to give you a continuous energy boost throughout the day. Choose complex carbohydrates that have fiber to slow digestion—these provide a steady flow of energy to help you feel like you can handle any challenge. Whole grains, fruits, and vegetables are fiber-filled, so they will keep you healthy while providing energy. Choose whole-grain breakfast cereals (like Total, Raisin Bran, and oatmeal), whole-wheat breads, brown rice, whole-wheat pastas, and fruits and vegetables.

Avoid sugary sweets (such as candies and cookies) and refined carbohydrates (such as white bread, white pasta, and white rice). They give you an energy high followed by a crash that leaves you feeling completely drained. These energy-robbing foods can exacerbate already rising stress levels. When you experience the energy crash, you are more likely to fall prey to cravings.

PROTEIN

Lately, the media has glamorized high-protein diets, claiming they build muscle and melt away fat. Exercise, not a high-protein diet, is required for building muscles and burning fat. The truth is that most of us have too much protein in our diets, and we're still fighting the fat war.

Protein is also responsible for helping your blood clot. It helps maintain the body's acid-base balance, which is critical. If the blood gets either too acidic or too basic, your bodily functions break down. The one thing your busy little protein is *not* designed to do is provide your body with energy, as many people think.

Protein is found in eggs, meat, poultry, and fish. Soybeans and their products, such as tofu and soymilk, are also good sources of protein. Remember, carbohydrates, such as beans and dairy products, do double duty as protein, as do nuts and seeds, which provide substantial amounts of protein but are considered fats.

FATS

Though fat has been the fall guy for America's growing weight problems, the truth is, fat is only trouble when you eat too much of it. In fact, fat is a vital component to every cell in your body—not just fat cells.

Fat, like protein, wears several metabolic hats. Fat not only supports and cushions your organs but also helps control blood pressure and blood clotting, and helps your body absorb the very important fat-soluble vitamins. Fat in your diet prevents your skin from becoming too dry, scaly, and lifeless.

Like nuts and seeds, oils, cream, butter, olives, mayonnaise, salad dressings, and avocados are considered fats. While all animal products—such as meat, fish, and poultry—and all dairy products (without the fat removed) contain fat, they are considered proteins. Likewise sweets, such as cookies and cakes, often have a lot of added fat, but you will find sweets on the carbohydrate lists. Just remember that like eating too much protein, gorging on fat will cause you to feel extremely sluggish. Much of your blood and oxygen supply will be diverted from the brain and muscles, where they are needed to rev up your metabolism, to your stomach to break down all the fat sitting there. While fats keep your metabolism speedy, some fats are better than others. I know it's bad to play favorites, but the fact is, some fats are heart healthy (unsaturated fats) and some (such as trans-fats and saturated fats) are not. So watch the potato chips and dips and fast foods.

STRESS AND EATING

Stress rarely takes a day off, and sometimes, despite all your good intentions, regular exercise, plenty of rest, and proper nutrition fall by the wayside. Eating right is the last thing on your mind when wedding plans go wrong. Ironically, it is times like this—when we wish we had "less on our plate"—that we have to watch what is actually on our plate.

Stressful conditions cause your stress hormone cortisol to rise. This may lead to intense cravings for fats and carbs, which can obviously lead to weight gain. However, by eating a balanced diet and preventing peaks and valleys in your energy level, you can keep your stress levels down and stop this vicious cycle of anxiety-induced appetite. When food shopping or dining out, keep the following in mind:

Be sure to get your Bs: B vitamins release energy from food—this is especially important when your body is in overdrive. Stress, both emotional and physical, causes the body to need more energy. Overlooking the increased need for B vitamins during times of stress can create vitamin deficiencies and leave you run-down. Good sources of B vitamins are leafy green veggies, potatoes, bananas, nuts, sunflower seeds, whole-grain breads, enriched cereals, pasta, peas, and fish.

Limit alcohol: I know, the first thing we want after interviewing bands, organizing the seating chart, or addressing the invitations once again is a drink, but it often does more harm than good. More than one or two glasses at a sitting can cause you to lose important B vitamins, affecting your immune system. Since alcohol acts as a depressant, slowing normal body functions, it adds additional stress to your body. You can't get as much done and your frustration level builds.

Watch your caffeine intake: One cup of coffee or one can of soda is okay for most adults, but too much can inhibit mineral absorption. Like alcohol, it adds stress to your entire system, causing your body to lose the minerals it needs for good health. I know it sounds like I am robbing you of your entire dietary support system, but a low to moderate intake of caffeine (and alcohol) coupled with a good balance of vitamins and minerals is a more enduring solution than a triple mocha latte or three apple martinis.

Drink the recommended eight 8-ounce glasses of water a day:
Water is essential to exercise and nutrition. Dehydration causes fatigue. Every process in your body is relying on water, and without enough of it, you can't function at your peak. When you are dehydrated, your stress can be exacerbated by afternoon headaches and sluggishness caused by dehydration.

Keep healthy snacks on hand: When we're hungry, we tend to reach for what's fast and easy. So it doesn't help when the refrigerator is stocked with ice cream. Start by making healthier choices as convenient as junk food. When you get home from the market with a bag of groceries, wash and trim those fresh veggies right away, keeping them within easy reach in the fridge. That way, the next time you crave something crunchy, you can choose from a platter of ready-to-eat carrots, celery, green beans, and whatever else you love to munch on.

WHAT ABOUT DIETARY AIDS?

Some dietary aids will help you maintain a healthy diet. I am not a fan of dietary aids because I believe most are dangerous and honestly don't work. I won't tell you not to take them (you're a grown-up and can decide for yourself) but if you do, make sure they support, not detract from, your fitness goals. For instance, what's the skinny on sports drinks, sports bars, and fat burners?

SPORTS DRINKS

Although sports drinks are very important for some athletes and can be beneficial for people who exercise for an hour and a half or more, 5 days a week, most people don't need them. In fact, for the average person who is trying to lose weight, sports drinks provide an extra source of calories and contribute to weight gain. Simply put, don't drink sports drinks if you are trying to lose weight unless regular, intense exercise is part of your normal routine.

Although convenient, these bars are usually the nutritional equivalent of candy-coated vitamins or candy bars with delusions of nutrition. You are much better off eating real food, like a piece of fruit and a couple of tablespoons of nuts. You'll get more fiber, vitamins, and minerals, and it will fill you up much more than the bar. Stick to the real food as much as possible.

FAT BURNERS

How many experts have said, "If there was a magic pill for weight loss, we'd all be thin!"? Most fat burners that work are more pill than magic, and they're banned in many areas. The others currently on the market are just a waste of money, as they do nothing for you. Eat healthfully and exercise—it's been proven to work. Stay away from the fat burners.

CALORIE COUNTING: DOES IT WORK?

I am not a big fan of calorie counting. Think about what you eat before you eat it. Chances are you know that stack of cookies or an extra dinner roll is not worth it, calorie-wise. In fact, being smart about calories, knowing in general the fat and sugar content of what you are eating, is a great step toward a healthier lifestyle. Besides, calorie counting to me is like following a budget; it's not much fun and I always wind up splurging.

SIZE COUNTS

We always think that bigger is better, but not when it comes to food servings. The misguided urgings of our parents to "clean our plates" and out-of-control restaurant portions often create a perfect storm of fat that lands right on our hips and thighs. Eating beyond feeling full or because you want to get your money's worth is an unhealthy standard in any reality. Now, while it's easy to understand why so many of us chronically overeat, the solution is even easier: portion control. Okay . . . have you stopped laughing? I am serious. In this case, you have to put less in it to win it—the war on weight gain, I mean.

First, you don't always have to eat everything that's put in front of you. Leaving the table a little hungry is not only smart eating; it makes you look refined and dainty. Start your education by measuring out portion sizes a few times so you get accustomed to how they look on your dishes. You can also use visual metaphors to help you. For example, one serving of pasta is about the size of a tennis ball, and one serving of meat is about the size of a deck of cards. When you're cooking at home, limit each plate to just one portion, and immediately put leftovers in a storage container. When eating out, ask your server to box half your meal to take home. Watching what you eat doesn't have to be an exercise in deprivation. Minor adjustments to your cooking and consumption will have the cumulative effect of weight loss and better health. And that's what's important. Use this chapter, as well as the next, to establish a commitment to lifelong fitness. And though what we should eat and how much seems to change with the season, never be discouraged. A well-balanced diet is within your reach, and fitness is a gift you can share.

True, much of this seems like common sense, but with the wedding fast approaching, anxiety begins to spike. I will show you how managing the mounting tension and keeping your relationship fit can burn calories and reignite passion.

CHAPTER 7

*Keeping
it
Off*

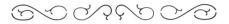

The beautiful princess and the lucky prince left the wedding to the cheers of family and friends. Flushed with champagne, food, and gifts, they looked forward to a life together full of health and fitness. All was grand and good until a year later, when our newlywed wanted to wear her dress from the rehearsal dinner for their first anniversary. With horror, she found that some witch—possibly his ex-girlfriend—had placed an evil curse on her and she couldn't zip it up. And worse, she now had a belly where none was before!

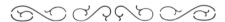

Okay, maybe this is a fairy tale, but as your fairy godtrainer, the best advice I can give the newly married is don't turn into couch potatoes! Statistics show marriage can make you fat. I'm serious! During the first year of marriage, women gain 1 ounce on their left ring finger and 10 or more pounds everywhere else. Don't let this happen to you. So how can you live "fitfully" ever after?

A HEALTHY LIFESTYLE AFTER THE WEDDING

While I don't expect you to follow the guidelines in this book during your reception, or even on your honeymoon (and those cruises can wreak havoc on your diet), you *can* use this chapter to establish a commitment to lifelong fitness. During the maintenance phase, weight loss is no longer the major motivator to stay active. But it is critical to keep up your routine because regular physical activity has been shown to be a contributing factor in the success of weight maintenance. And let's face it—you worked hard to get here. Do you want to have to do it all over again?

If you're serious about keeping the weight off, you need to be serious about your workouts. Keep your activity level high, both in and out of the gym. Your workouts should consist of both cardiovascular training and strength training. But how much exercise is necessary? Your cardiovascular exercise should still be done 3 to 5 times per week at moderate to high intensity. Your strength training should be done 3 to 4 times per week, and you should do some stretching every day.

Pardon the pun, but you won't stay married to any one program (including this one). Vary your exercise programs and keep your muscles guessing. With so many programs out there, you are bound to fall in love with something new. Have you tried Kettlebells yet? What about TRX? Not familiar? It's suspension training using a tool designed for this workout that leverages gravity and your body weight to perform hundreds of exercises. It's awesome and a whole lot of fun. My new favorites are hot yoga and TurboFire, a kick boxing program designed by Chalene Johnson for Beachbody. You can order it at www.beachbody.com. For more ideas, e-mail me at BonneMarcus@gmail.com.

DIET STRATEGIES

With regard to diet, don't throw everything you've learned out the window right after the big day! Sorry—you can't go back to eating at the drive-through and expect to maintain your weight loss. Here are some simple things you can do to avoid sabotaging all that hard work:

Stock your fridge with healthy foods so that when you get the urge to munch, you are surrounded by nourishing foods that will help you, not hurt.

Don't wait more than 4 hours between meals and don't skip meals—this will only set you up for binging and consuming excess calories.

Keep calories low. Gone are the days of eating mindlessly. Be aware of everything that goes into your mouth, whether by journaling or simply keeping a mental tally.

Avoid sugary foods, which will cause energy highs followed by crashes. These crashes signal your body to get more fuel quickly, and so you turn to more sugar for a quick pick-me-up.

Eat plenty of fiber-rich foods, like fruits, veggies, and beans. The fiber will help fill you up so that you feel satiated.

Don't deny yourself your favorite foods. Allow yourself to have small planned portions every now and then so that you don't feel deprived and you don't end up bingeing.

TRACK YOURSELF

Your biggest fear is gaining back weight, but don't be afraid of your scale. Weigh yourself at least once each week to monitor any gains. If the numbers begin to climb, then reduce calories and increase your exercise.

ACCEPT SETBACKS

No one is perfect—not even you! If you miss your workout one day or binge on a bag of Fritos it's not that big a deal. It happens. If you slip up, do not beat yourself up over it. Simply get back to your healthy lifestyle rather than letting yourself backslide into your old habits.

The bad news is that 90 to 95 percent of those who lose weight will be unsuccessful at keeping the weight off. Do not be a statistic. Nothing feels as good as losing weight and living in the body you've always dreamed of. And who knows? Maybe being fit and trim will help you have a happier marriage. Did you know sweat can actually bring the two of you closer? How? Working out produces endorphins, and endorphins give you that exercise high. When you exercise together and both produce these endorphins, you end up associating those positive feelings with your partner.

Keep in mind that a difference in fitness ability may cause frustration for both of you, so find a compromise. If you're more fit than your partner, be the role model. Give encouraging words. Use healthy competition. For example, if you both enjoy running, allow the person who is going slower to initially set the pace. You will still be getting a good workout. You'll be working in your target heart-rate zone and burning calories. Eventually you're both going to get to the same level. If he's the one who's more fit, understand that, and after you set the pace at the beginning of the run and enjoy some time running together, let him go ahead.

Despite the benefits of working out together, there are still days when you will get a better workout on your own. Unfortunately, just because you and your honey get along in life doesn't mean you're compatible as exercise buddies. If there's a great disparity in your fitness levels, experiences, or temperaments, or if you find you're too competitive to share any activity, don't push it. Just work out separately around the same time in the gym. With your blood pumping and bodies glistening, it's good to remember that you can always meet up later for a shower.

Want to reap the benefits of a couples workout? Here are some suggestions: Level the playing field and begin a new workout together. Start something fresh for both of you, like a class in kickboxing, yoga, or weight training. You can support each other on this new adventure. What if one of you works out regularly and the other does not? In this case, exercising together will take a little creativity since an intense workout for one might be too easy for the other. To leap this exercise hurdle, you can:

Alternate weight training by spotting and encouraging each other. Adjust the weight and intensity that's right for you and for him.

Find low-impact activities you can enjoy together that improve fitness daily. We sometimes think we'll save walking for when we can't workout anymore, but it provides excellent health benefits. And the opportunity for long talks is great for any relationship.

Start with a 20-minute walk 3 to 5 times a week, working up to walking 3 miles 5 to 6 times a week. Take it slow. Increase distance by no more than 10 percent each week.

Make plans to do something special that incorporates exercise, perhaps a dance class or a hike in the mountains.

Having fitness as a common pursuit will not only keep you exercising; it will help you maintain a better diet. This can lead to increased self-esteem and more energy to do and share other things. If you respect each other's individual needs and goals, working out with your sweetie can only do you good, both individually and as a couple. So get out there and enjoy it together. My best guess is that once you embrace the tips in this book, you'll want to embrace each other far more often!

CHAPTER 8

Wedding Stress Solutions

By their very nature, weddings are stress-producing events. One minute you are ebullient and the next you can't stand your fiancé and you just don't know why. Much of the stress comes from all the details you have to manage, coupled with the feeling that you have no control over all that's going on. The best advice given to me came from my twin sister, who is a social worker. She said, "Remember, it is about getting married to the man you love, not about the huge party you are throwing for two hundred of your closest friends."

As a trainer, I know there is more to exercise than just getting in shape physically. Exercise helps to reduce stress. And who wouldn't be stressed planning her dream wedding? You are always encouraged to get advice from wedding professionals; I recommend you try some of my favorite fitness solutions as well.

STRESSOR # 1: BUDGET PLANNING

For most brides-to-be, setting the budget is the biggest stress factor in wedding planning. You like to think you can keep money matters in perspective, but I remember the fights with my groom when we decided to pay for our wedding. We wanted to treat our near and dear to a feast, including a full bar and a Venetian hour. However, the quality of the meal had a direct impact on the size of the guest list. While we narrowed our list down to a mere 175 people, it was still too many for me. My groom's immediate family was close to 120 people, while my immediate family and friends barely totaled 50. We argued over inviting my personal trainer (yes, I had a trainer too) as opposed to some of his cousins. No matter how many we invited to the wedding, there always seemed to be someone we'd forgotten. Then the stress was compounded by guilt. I had a traditional Jewish wedding, after all.

But, budget planning is like working out; you avoid problems by writing everything down and learning to make adjustments as you go along. Modify your budget as you move from engagement to reception.

Be selective in what *you must have* and what you can afford. Arguments over ordering top-shelf liquor versus orchids in your flower arrangements should not detract from the reasons you're getting married.

Here's a way to cope when the fighting begins. Put down the calculator and checkbook and go for a nice, long run outdoors.

RUN AWAY FROM YOUR PROBLEMS

Fresh air: what a concept! Running is a workout you can take anywhere. There's just something soothing about the rhythm of your breathing and your feet hitting the ground. Running gives you a chance to think, to put some distance, emotionally, between you and the stresses of your wedding. Running triggers the release of endorphins, natural chemicals that ease the pain and elevate your mood (what some people call a "runner's high").

To make it even better, invite your fiancé along. (See Chapter 6 on Keeping it Off) Running with your fiancé will invigorate your daily life and create a support system for achieving health-related goals, both physical and social. It will strengthen your bodies and your relationship. A good pair of shoes and a supportive sports bra are all you need.

■ *Sports Bra*

There are two main categories of sports bra: compression and encapsulation. For most women, the compression bra is fine. It works by compressing the breasts against the chest and holding them in place so they have limited mobility. The encapsulation sports bra works by supporting each individual breast against the chest. It's a better choice for the larger-breasted woman. Whichever bra you choose, be sure to try it on before purchasing it. You'll be more active in it than a regular bra, so you'll want to make sure it fits properly. My personal favorite is the Lululemon Booby Bracer bra.

■ *Sneakers*

Choosing the right shoe reduces your chances for injuries and can make running (or any workout you choose) more effective and more enjoyable. Your feet and ankles need a certain degree of support, stability, and flexibility while still offering the proper cushioning to protect your joints. Because feet are unique to each individual, you may need extra room in the forefoot, a tighter heel, and/or stronger arch support. Running sneakers should be lightweight with plenty of cushioning for shock absorption, stability, forefoot flexibility, and traction. My current favorite is New Balance. What works for me may not be right for you, so I recommend visiting a store that specializes in running shoes, getting measured and trying on a few different brands.

TIPS FOR BEGINNERS

Start slowly. You'll have fewer problems with sore muscles or other injuries if you don't work too hard the first few days or even the first few weeks. You'll enjoy running more if you try to do less than you're capable of. You'll also achieve more, since the most important factor in achieving success is consistency. The best approach for beginners is to start by walking briskly for 30 minutes, 3 times a week, for 2 weeks. Then, insert short jogging distances during the walk. It is important to go at your own pace; that is, listen to your body. You build endurance by working out longer. Increase your body's capacity to stay in motion and before you know it, you're running 3 to 4 miles with ease.

TIPS ON FORM

Running requires some instruction. Things like focus on good posture, look ahead as you run, and not down at the ground. My running hero Stu Mittleman, author of *Slow Burn*, offers the following tips related to form:

" 1. When you move, bring your arms up into dinosaur arm position. Picture a *Tyrannosaurus rex*, with tiny little arms that remain bent at the elbow. This is the position you want your arms to be in.

2. Next, imagine you are holding a butterfly in each hand. Your hands are closed around the butterfly just enough to keep

them from flying away. Relax your hands enough so that the butterfly has room to flutter its wings.

3. Imagine you are standing on top of the world as it is rotating. Lift your feet up just enough to let the earth pass beneath you."

PUT YOUR BEST FOOT FORWARD

Strength training the muscles you use for running will improve your overall performance and decrease your chance of getting injured. Too much mileage too soon can put stress on tendons and muscles. Running creates a force 3.5 to 8 times your body weight on impact, so your feet really take a beating. You can prevent shin splints (which are sometimes caused by an imbalance in the muscles of the lower leg) by strengthening the tibialis anterior (shin) and stretching the calves. Incorporate the following exercises to avoid muscle imbalances in your lower legs.

Toe taps: Sit in a chair with your feet flat on the floor, and place your ankles directly below your knees. Keep your feet parallel and hip-width apart. Press into your heels and raise your toes toward your knees. Perform fast toe taps until you feel fatigue in the lower legs. Do approximately 25 to 35 taps. Work up to 2 sets with a 30-second rest between sets.

Alphabet: This is my name for another exercise I recommend. Sit in a chair with one foot flat on the floor and the other leg extended and off the floor. With your lifted foot, point your toes and "draw" the letters of the alphabet from A to Z. It sounds silly, but try it.

Towel pull: Sit on a chair with your feet flat on the floor; place a bath towel on the floor under your right foot. Beginning at one end of the towel, use your toes to grab the towel, pulling it back toward you. Keep working this way from one end of the towel to the other. When you finish, repeat with the left foot.

MOTIVATIONAL TIPS

Don't despair. Occasional lack of motivation strikes even the most disciplined runners. Try to remember how good you felt about yourself after completing your last run and be proud that you've started a program at all. Then, follow these handy tips to keep yourself going.

1. Buy something new.
My personal favorite. New athletic shoes may be just the jump-start you need. Shopping always works for me. If your outsoles look worn and the arch is drooping, it's time to shop. Most experts recommend at least one new pair a year. Remember, supportive, comfortable shoes are imperative to the health of your feet, ankles, and knees.

2. Tune up.
Download your favorite "get moving" music and go running with headphones.

3. Location inspiration.
Break up the monotony by trying different routes. Explore new areas in your town or drive to a park, beach, or new neighborhood for a change of scenery.

4. Vary your intensity.
Vary speed and intensity to stay focused and build endurance and strength. Mix running on flat ground with walking uphill, or try running fast for 20 seconds or longer and then jogging slowly to catch your breath.

5. Make running philanthropic.
AIDS Walks, Race for the Cure, or local fun runs are great events to keep you training, and they often have local clubs that will help you design a fitness plan. There are also charity apps that make

exercising philanthropic while you train for those bigger events. Visit www.charitymiles.org.

6. Make running appointments.

Make a running schedule and stick to it. Write down the days to run, how far to go, and which route to take. Once your schedule is in writing, you're more likely to do it. If running is not for you, here are the top 10 reasons why walking is a great alternative.

1. You can walk anywhere and everywhere. Go sightseeing in your own city.

2. Anybody can do it. No coordination required. Unlike aerobic classes, a popular non-running form of exercise that may leave you scheming to sneak out early, walking is "natural," since we all walk upright by design.

3. Walking promotes bone health. Walking places regular impact on the joints, which helps prevent both osteoporosis and osteoarthritis. Walk today so you can walk taller tomorrow.

4. Walking is a low-impact activity allowing walkers to enjoy a relatively low injury rate.

5. Walking tones the butt and thighs. Add an incline to your treadmill workout or walk on hilly terrain to sculpt the derriere and burn a few extra calories.

6. Walking boosts energy levels. A good ten-minute walk is better than a cup of coffee during that low-energy dip in the workday. Looking for change for the vending machine around 3 p.m.? Craving a sugary snack to wake you up? Skip it and take a brisk walk.

7. Motion changes emotion. Feeling depressed or overwhelmed? Then get your body moving. Walking eliminates stress hormones (catecholamines) in the body and reduces tension in your butt, gut, thighs, and calves.

8. Walking sheds pounds and inches. Shouldn't this be the number-one reason?

9. Walking can be a social event or spark your love life. Walking groups give you the chance to see friends, have heart-to-heart talks and get encouragement. Invite your fiancé to join in a romantic moonlight walk along the beach to ignite further calorie-burning activities later on.

10. Walking increases the production of beta-endorphins, hormones that calm the body and prepare it for restful sleep.

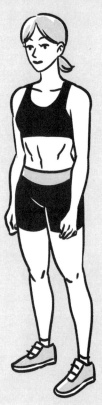

Whether you decide to walk or run, maximize the effectiveness of your workout by remembering preparation and reparation. Proper warm-up and stretching (See Chapter 1 on Getting Started), before and after your walk, will insure every step you take will be a safe and healthy one.

STRESSOR #2:
OVERWHELMING DETAILS

Ordering the invitations; finding the photographer, the caterer, the florists, the baker; and securing the out-of-town guest hotel reservations . . . Where does it end?

GET CENTERED!

Pilates is an exercise in mind–body connection that will help get you centered, reducing stress and allowing you to better focus on all the details of wedding planning. Joseph Pilates called his practice Contrology, defined as "the harmonious melding of the body, the mind, and the spirit."

The Pilates system created by Joseph Pilates is a form, like ballet. The method evolved out of Pilates's interest in overcoming illness and becoming physically stronger. Much of the Pilates system references his training in fitness and sports, as well as his work in the circus and as a self-defense trainer. You step inside the form, and through a consistent practice you gain an understanding of how to work within the structure. Through a series of non–weight bearing exercises performed on a mat and five pieces of uniquely designed equipment, you gain a strong, supple, and energized body, mind, and spirit.

The first requirement is concentration; the mind is attuned to the body. Through a series of exercises that emphasize alignment, precision, and breath, you flow from one exercise to the next (like a dance sequence) steadily gaining strength, flexibility, balance, and overall control of the body. The focal point of the work is to strengthen the "powerhouse," or the central region of the body that includes the abdomen, the lower back, and buttock area. A strong powerhouse provides the core support to master the wide variety of exercises in the Pilates system. There are hundreds of exercises from which to create a system tailored to your needs, and *boredom* is not in the Pilates vocabulary. The best perk of all is that you walk away with a practice you can do on your own anywhere you are: at home, in the gym, or even on the beach!

Besides bridesmaids not living up to their duties, I believe the number-one conflict associated with bridesmaids is what they will wear. One of your bridesmaids is a petite size 4 and the other a healthy size 12. How do you select a dress that will make them both feel comfortable? Can you also put them both in a seafoam green dress with Kermit the Frog green embroidery? If they love you, then the answer is yes.

GROUP FITNESS WILL BRING YOU TOGETHER

Seriously, the dress dilemma is much more common than you may realize. Other conflicts can also arise between you and your bridesmaids. I know I felt a little neglected by one or two of my bridesmaids, but what can you do? You should not allow your attendants to make you miserable. After all, you have asked those closest to you to share in your happiness. Besides, with all of the details involved in planning a wedding, you certainly don't need the added stress. So, if you have bridesmaids that have different physiques, modesty and simplicity are two factors you might consider in selecting the bridesmaid dress. You can counteract or solve any disputes over dresses or partners (no one may want to be paired with the usher with the comb-over) by organizing workout activities with your bridesmaids.

Group activities for the bride and her attendants shouldn't be confined to a bachelorette field trip to a strip club. Trying exercise classes together will be fun and a great bonding opportunity. You can schedule a different workout class once a week. Believe me, there is no shortage of fitness classes to choose from.

BOSU INTEGRATED TRAINING

When working out on a stable surface, gravity supports you but limits the amount of muscle firing during your workout. BOSU boot camp takes that support system out of the equation and gravitational force is used to one's advantage! Olympians and elite athletes from a variety of sports have experienced the benefits of BOSU (pronounced BOW like the thing they put on your wedding gift and SUE like don't sue me for not giving you the right gift) by incorporating it into their strength and conditioning training. BOSU boot camp is designed around the unique BOSU balance trainer. BOSU, an acronym for "both sides up," is named for the unit's special ability to be flipped during the workout, revealing different surfaces, each with its own advantages. With one side a twelve-inch vinyl dome inflated to a height of twelve inches and the other side a twenty-five-inch-wide flat platform, this apparatus provides for intense cardiovascular, strength training, and core exercises.

BOSU boot camp challenges participants by constantly changing one's center of gravity, providing a workout that develops incredible levels of core stability and balance. Participants of all fitness levels can participate in the boot camp. In fact, just stepping on and off the BOSU will immediately reap rewards of increased body awareness and balance. The class exercises include lunges, squats, cardiovascular activity, abdominal work, push-ups, and triceps extensions. Each exercise can be modified and performed to accommodate any fitness level.

CARDIO STRIPTEASE

When working out at the gym, you expect to shed pounds—but clothing? Cardio Striptease has everybody talking and gawking! Fusing fitness and entertainment, Cardio Striptease involves building confidence through sexuality and empowering, erotic, athletic exercises. This is a very stylized form of dance that embraces the physical body in terms of the sexual body. Dance movements are choreographed to specific music designed to get the body pumping. A 10-minute warm-up introduces basic movements, isolations, and techniques followed by static stretching. Participants learn the art of pole dancing, making an entrance, turning, gyrating, body language, throwing attitude, flirting, posing, and the use of props. For the last 25 minutes of class, participants perform a choreographed striptease. Routines feature music and dance movements with erotic undertones. Removing articles of clothing is optional. I suggest saving that for the honeymoon.

If you've ever wondered about all those odd-looking straps hanging in your gym, let me share more about working out with them. It may have been developed for the Navy SEALs, but it's beginner-friendly and designed for anyone. The concept of the TRX suspension training is pretty basic: You use two straps on your feet or hands to partially suspend your body and use your own body weight as resistance.

The muscle groups you work, as well as how hard you work them, all depend on the positioning of your body on the cables. You're in control of how much you want to challenge yourself on each exercise—because you can simply adjust your body position to add or decrease resistance. You can do it all with TRX, from lunges to planks to upper body resistance exercises. And the best part? Your workouts can change as many times as you want them to. That means that both your mind and your body will stay challenged with all the ways you can mix up your workouts.

If you've never done TRX, sign up for a class at your gym, if they offer one, before you commit to any at-home or individual training. That way your instructor can teach you the proper way to do a move without injuring yourself.

Zumba is now being taught at over fifty thousand locations in seventy-five countries, with an astonishing six million participants taking classes every week. Why? It's a workout camouflaged as a dance party. Created by celebrity fitness trainer Alberto "Beto" Perez in the mid-'90s, Zumba combines easy-to-follow routines with the Latin rhythms of salsa, merengue, hip-hop, and more that will blow you away. Zumba is the kind of cardio workout that makes it easy and fun to get in shape. The best part is that you don't even need to know how to dance.

STRESSOR # 4:
DIVORCED PARENTS

When your parents are divorced and aren't talking except when they're arguing, feeling like a negotiator can add to your already escalating prewedding stress levels.

CARRY THEM TO THEIR SEPARATE CORNERS

Pumping iron is always the best way to relieve stress, and in the process, you develop the strength to carry your parents to their neutral corners.

There are benefits to lifting weights that have been covered in Chapter 1. But just a reminder: Lifting weights allows muscles to work in a manner that resembles real-life movements. (Embracing your fiancé uses the biceps, pectorals, and anterior deltoids, and done right, can lead to using the abdominal and adductor muscles.) Free weights integrate more muscle into a movement. You require several muscles to move, balance, and steady the body as you lift and lower a weight. For me, any activity that keeps your bones healthy, helps control your weight, decreases your resting blood pressure (which may elevate due to parental interference) and boosts your energy has to make you a happier, more productive person. Of course, hoisting hunks of steel is not an instant cure-all, but you'd be surprised how much satisfaction a pair of 20-pound dumbbells can bring into your life.

STRESSOR # 5:
UNSOLICITED OPINIONS

Too many opinions from too many people may have you wanting to buy noise-canceling earphones or industrial-strength duct tape. But you don't have to go to those extremes, even though you might want to.

A 20-minute yoga time-out is just the answer. Whether you are looking for a way to change your workout or your mind-body connection, yoga may be just the thing you need. Here is a mini workout that will have you "blissed out" and planning your honeymoon to India by the end of the week! Or maybe just feeling really great and ready for more . . .

Before you begin, prep your space to achieve maximum yoga results and find the perfect attire to ensure comfort and mobility. Hardwood floors are preferred over carpet, and bare feet are a must. It is nice to have a yoga mat, but it is not required. Little touches such as candles and incense set the mood. Music can also be a nice addition to your yoga practice. Your regular workout clothes are fine for yoga practice. Sometimes a pair of loose pants and a form fitted top is okay, so long as it isn't constricting/restricting, but by no means are they required. The most important thing is that you are comfy and unrestricted.

Now you're ready to bust some yoga moves!

Sun salutations are the basis for most Vinyasa yoga classes. Sun salutation, or Surya Namaskar as they are called in Sanskrit, create heat in the body and get all the major muscle groups moving. They can be practiced alone or as part of a longer practice/class. You can also use sun salutations as part of your regular fitness routine. There are many variations of the sun salutation. Here is a variation called Sun Salutation A.

Start by standing with your feet together and your hands together in prayer in front of your heart in Mountain pose. Feel all four corners of your feet reaching down into the earth as if your feet are rooting into the ground. Feel the inner leg lift from the arches of the feet all the way up the body and out through the crown of the head. Feel the neck lengthen, lift the heart center, and allow the sacrum (tailbone) to drop.

Close your eyes and take 5 slow inhalations and exhalations. If your body is a bit wobbly, you can slightly separate the feet. Continue to breathe. After 5 breaths, open your eyes. You are now ready to begin.

Now stand in Mountain pose and reconnect the feet into the floor. Lengthen the spine and lift the heart. Inhale, sweep the arms out to your sides and up into a long-armed prayer. The back of the neck is long. Lift your gaze toward your thumbs without crunching the back of the neck. Exhale, then bend at the waist while swan-diving the arms over the legs, bringing the hands to the floor. Release the back of the neck. This is the Standing Forward Bend.

If the hands don't reach the floor, you can place them on your thighs or shins. Inhale, resting the fingertips in front of the toe tips, then lift the gaze, coming into Flat Back position. Lengthen from navel to nose. If the fingertips don't reach the floor, you can place the palms on your shins or thighs. Exhale, lunge your right leg back with the toes tucked.

Next, inhale and lunge your left leg back to meet the right leg, coming into a plank position. Exhale, bend the elbows straight back toward your heels (doing a push-up in plank position) and lower into Four-Limbed Staff Pose. You want to keep the body from touching the floor, but by no means should you force yourself to hold a bent-arm position if it is really uncomfortable. If simply softening the elbows is enough for you, that is fine.

Inhale, straighten the arms, and drop the hips and legs toward the floor in Upward Facing Dog pose. Ideally, only the palms of the hands and the tops of the feet touch the floor. Again, if this is uncomfortable, keep the thighs on the floor and slowly work toward lifting them up.

Exhale, roll over the feet, and lift your hips up and back as if you are trying to touch them to the wall behind you, your rear in the air and your head down, in Downward Facing Dog pose. Slide the shoulder blades up the back. Lengthen the hips away from the waist. Press the thigh muscles back and reach the calves to the floor. It's okay if the heels do not touch the floor. Take 3 to 5 deep breaths in Downward Dog.

Inhale, lift your eyes, and gaze between your hands. Scoop out the belly and come high onto the balls of the feet. Exhale, step your feet one at a time between your hands. Inhale into Flat Back position. Exhale to Standing Forward Bend.

Inhale and sweep the arms out and up, reversing the swan dive into a long-armed prayer pose. Exhale, bringing the hands in front of the heart into Mountain pose. Repeat this sequence 3 to 5 times and, before you know it, you're wedding stress will have melted away.

If there is a wedding stressor that I haven't covered, please e-mail me at BonneMarcus@gmail.com. I will definitely have an answer for you.

Frequently Asked Questions

With this book I have tried to inform and support you. It is important to me to give you everything you need to be successful. So please review some of the most frequently asked questions, common fitness mistakes, and myths so that you can easily avoid them.

HEALTH AND FITNESS ARE NOT THE SAME

This common misconception—health equals fitness—affects why and how you exercise, and it is probably the source of much frustration. "I work out religiously and still can't lose those last ten pounds!" If I had a dollar every time a client has made that complaint . . .

To be clear, *health* is defined as the state where all the systems of the body—nervous, muscular, skeletal, circulatory, lymphatic, etc.—are working in an optimal way. *Fitness* is the physical ability to perform athletic activity. For example, are you running to get in shape (health) or to compete in a marathon (fitness)? You don't have to choose between health and fitness, but always put your health first if you wish to achieve lasting physical fitness.

WHAT BRIDES WANT TO KNOW

Over the years, I have tried to "marry" the emotional needs of the women I train to their physical realities. I pride myself not just on training young women, but also on educating them in a way that insures good health and fitness. Here are a few of the most common, and thereby the most valuable, questions and answers. Any of them strike a chord?

Six months is a reasonable amount of time to lose ten pounds, so following a liquid diet or worse, starving yourself, is not recommended. Not eating enough or starvation WILL result in weight loss. So will chopping off a body part, which makes about as much sense. The problem with severely reducing caloric intake is that once your body realizes it is being starved, it will literally hold on to stored fat and refuse to let it go. The body then begins to use other stored nutrients to fuel activity, namely protein. Once this occurs, muscle mass decreases and so does metabolism.

The best and most lasting means of losing weight is to eat healthfully—cut back on calories without sacrificing nutrition (see Chapter 5, The Bride's Healthy-Eating Guide)—and exercise regularly. It's simple math, really: If you trim a few hundred calories off your daily intake and burn a few hundred calories through exercise, you can lose a pound or two per week, depending on your height and your starting weight.

First understand that there are two types of exercise: aerobic (a.k.a. cardio) and strength-building. Doing only aerobics is a big no-no. Aerobic exercise is wonderful . . . it strengthens the heart and lungs, burns calories, and there is nothing like a jog through the park on a sunny day. But in and of itself, it is not enough. Next time you are at the health club, take a look at the women who do nothing but aerobic exercise. Then take a look at the women who are spending time lifting weights. Women who correctly incorporate strength training in addition to cardiovascular exercise not only have better-looking bodies, but they are also stronger and tend to have a lower percentage of body fat.

Next, stop worrying about bulking up. Only about 10 percent of women will build large muscles, and that's due to genetics. If you are one of the 10 percent and don't want to gain muscle bulk, concentrate on high repetitions with low weight and variety in your aerobic exercise routine. Focus on how good exercise makes you feel, not how you would like to look. Accept your body for what it is and not on other standards.

3. I was thinking of buying the Torso Track or the AB-DOer. Do you think these are good machines?

The abominable abdominal machine is my favorite question. It seems as if every week on late-night TV there's a new infomercial selling yet another device "guaranteed to flatten your abs in just a few short weeks." In a moment of weakness, you pull out your Visa and purchase the "gut-busting contraption." It arrives and you try it a few times. Eventually it ends up in the infomercial-gadget graveyard collecting dust in your closet. Sound familiar?

You do not need a fancy abdominal product to get a defined middle. And the only spot reduction available for the abdominal area is called liposuction. Abdominal exercises alone are not effective for gaining dynamite definition. Abdominal exercises strengthen the muscles, but they don't burn the fat off the muscles. Keep in mind there's no substitute for hard work and commitment.

4. Do those neoprene suits help you lose weight?

Wearing too many clothes or plastic neoprene sweat suits with the belief it will help you lose weight is not only foolish, it is VERY dangerous. When you work out, your body turns up the heat. Your muscles are like little furnaces, thermodynamically converting calories into energy to fuel your effort. And you get hot. As that happens, your body has to maintain your core temperature to keep your internal organs cool, so it generates sweat that evaporates off your skin and naturally cools your body. Mother Nature creates this miracle of efficiency in our bodies. It is not nice to fool with Mother Nature by wearing these less-than-fashionable neoprene sweat suits. You generate more heat, which in turn, generates more sweat. You will absolutely lose weight. The weight you will lose is water. Ultimately you will be in a dehydrated state for up to 48 hours.

5. When I drop a few pounds, it always seems to come off my face or my chest—never my thighs or my butt. Are there any exercises I can do to burn fat where I actually want it burned?

It's a myth to say that you can decide where you want to lose fat. The only way to spot reduce is called liposuction. I recommend weight training. In combination with regular aerobic exercise (which burns fat all over), weight training can help you change the shape of your body—within the limitations of your basic size and shape, of course. While you can't give yourself model-slim hips if you weren't born with them, it is possible to sculpt leaner legs, a more shapely rear, and defined arms.

6. I want to tone my arms so I look good in my sleeveless gown. Should I do more repetitions on my arm exercises or lift heavier weights?

Lifting weight, whether you do many repetitions or use a heavier weight, will certainly help your arms for a sleeveless dress. But if you have been lifting 8-pound dumbbells and find that you can do a ridiculous number of reps without getting tired, I would definitely recommend switching to a heavier weight. To build and tone, you have to stress muscles to the point at which they are completely exhausted; it's in the rest-and-repair period that your muscle gains strength. So if you breeze through your sets, or it takes many sets for your muscles to feel tired, you're not doing yourself much good. When you're training efficiently, your last reps should feel really hard, and you should not be able to do more without compromising proper form. But remember that toning the muscle is only part of the battle. If your muscles are camouflaged by a layer of body fat, make sure you are doing cardio exercises to burn fat so your newly sleek muscles will show.

7. I have a hard time sticking to my routine. I go to the gym and do exercise videos at home. I get so bored and always wimp out before seeing results! How can I get motivated?

Take time out to evaluate your current routine and create a new one. Of course, my workout is exciting enough to keep you challenged and motivated; but as I have said, you won't stay married to any one routine, including mine.

So when motivation flags, use the following guidelines to help you spring-clean your workout.

When in doubt, throw your workout out. Be honest, and assess if you truly stuck to your plan last year. How many workouts did you miss? Too many to count? Don't beat yourself up about a lack of follow through; instead, determine the reasons that influenced the breakdown. Perhaps you missed too many workouts because you didn't plan your schedule accordingly. Lack of planning is also a common reason for not following through. If that's the case, take out your appointment book and schedule them in. Maybe your present workout no longer excites you. Does it include strength training? Maybe substitute an hour on the treadmill with a step or Spinning class. Hiring a personal trainer is also a good way of staying motivated.

Reassess your goals. Take the time to analyze your efforts so you can meet the goals you set for yourself. Determine what changes you need to make and then implement strategies that will influence the results you want.

Cater your routine to your body. Working out is great for your body, unless your workout is causing injuries. That's why you should always know your physical limitations. For example, if you want to take up or continue running this year, then make sure your shoes cater to your feet. Those of us with fallen arches need a different support system in our shoes than those with bunions, and so on. Do you have a chronic condition such as diabetes, high blood pressure, or coronary artery disease? You need to create a workout that is compatible with your ability. You should never have to give up working out. Ask your doctor for help.

Seek help. This may be the perfect time to enlist the aid of a professional to help you jump-start your new workout in the right direction. Hire a qualified personal trainer for a few sessions to review your workout results. He or she can give you great ideas for more effective workouts or determine what needs to be changed to obtain greater results. If nutrition is the hard part for you, meet with a nutritionist for detailed eating plans based on your goals. I am always available and you can contact me at BonneMarcus@gmail.com for help.

9. I joined Weight Watchers, as well as my company's on-site gym. I have been working out, recording and watching what I eat. I have lost 10 pounds so far. I would like to lose an additional 40 for my wedding. I have heard and read a lot about Hydroxycut, and I am wondering what your opinion on that fat burner is. Do you think this would help speed up the weight loss?

First of all, congratulations on joining Weight Watchers and starting an exercise program. If you would like to know how I feel about products like Hydroxycut, I will sum it up in one word: Dangerous. Hydroxycut and products like it contain the ingredient ephedra, also called ma huang. Many people make the mistake of assuming these ingredients are safe because they are herbs, which they feel are all natural and harmless. However, ephedra use has resulted in heart attacks and strokes and even deaths! MetaboLife, Thermogenics Plus, and Ultra Diet Pep are a few of the many diet products that have ephedra in them. In addition to ephedra, they also may contain other caffeine-like substances. Stay away from products containing garcinia cambogia, aloe, senna, and buckthorn—these are either ineffective or harmful. I know you are in a hurry to lose weight, but my first concern is always health. You are already on the right path. Please continue without the use of these ergogenic aids.

A little knowledge will go a long way in your health-and-fitness program. Heed these basic cautions to help you on your way to a healthier body and soul.

In fitness and in health,
Bonne Marcus

RESOURCES

Here are a few extra sources for information about the techniques used in this book, plus fitness inspiration to help you on your journey. And remember, I'm always available to help you out with questions and concerns if you'd like to send me an email at BonneMarcus@gmail.com.

TECHNIQUE

Bosu.com: The official site for the BoSu system, this webpage includes training videos, workouts of the week, and even an app.

ExRx.net: This site includes detailed descriptions of over 1,600 different exercises, including animated GIFs depicting proper form for each one.

TRXtraining.com: Information on using TRX—very helpful!
Zumba.com: Zumba gear, videos, and information about where to Zumba.

EQUIPMENT

Collagevideo.com: A huge resource for workout videos in a wide variety of disciplines.

Lebertfitness.com: The homepage for Marc Lebert, creator of the Equalizer.

Lifefitness.com: The place for stationary bikes, elliptical machines, and treadmills.

Lululemon.com: My personal choice for stylish workout wear.

Performbetter.com: My favorite site overall for purchasing fitness equipment.

Spinning.com: Your one-stop shop for spinning bikes, gear, and information about facilities around the country where you can take spin classes.

INSPIRATION

Charitymiles.org: A great app for raising money for charities while you walk, run, or bike.

Myfitnesspal.com: Handy tools for calorie counting and a supportive community to back you up while you get fit.

Nutritiontwins.com: The homepage for Tammy Lakatos Shames and Elysse Lakatos, the Nutrition Twins!

Q.equinox.com: Q is the luxury gym chain Equinox's health blog, which includes a fun mix of exercise techniques and information from personal trainers, as well as articles on food, healthy living, fashion, and travel.

Wellandgood.com: *Well + Good* is an online magazine with great articles about fitness trends, plenty of recipes, and personal interviews with a wide variety of people about how they stay fit.

Worldultrafit.com: This is the homepage for ultra marathoner and athlete Stu Mittleman, author of *Slow Burn*.

HEALTH AND FITNESS DIARY

You can use the following pages to log your progress on the journey to fitness. For more information, see Chapter 2: Diary of a Fit Bride (page 16).

ACKNOWLEDGMENTS

This book would not have been possible without the support of my family and friends. I want to give a special thank you to Robert and Lisa Cincinnati, Stacey Martinez, Debra Melendez, and Vincent Marano for their time and generosity.

Additional thanks to Maddi-Lyn Alvarez for her endless energy and enthusiasm while modeling and my niece Jennifer Crow-Galarza who was the inspiration for this book.

Thank you to Tammy Lakatos Shames RDN, CDN, CFT and Lyssie Lakatos RDN, CDN, CFT aka "The Nutrition Twins" for providing their expertise. I owe special thanks to Sterling Publishing for "accepting my proposal" and providing an amazing team to work with. Thank you to my editor Kate Zimmermann for her guidance, patience, and support as well as Kim Broderick, production editor, Nina Matsumoto for her perfectly detailed illustrations, and Yeon Kim, for her exceptional book design.

Finally a special thank you to my loving husband and best friend Larry who always believed in me.

INDEX